ECG Complete

Dedication
This book is dedicated to our sons Luke and Nicki.

Commissioning Editor: Laurence Hunter
Development Editor: Janice Urquhart
Project Manager: Nancy Arnott
Design Direction: Erik Bigland
Illustrators: Gillian Lee, David Graham

ECG Complete

Steven Bowbrick BSc

Chief Cardiac Physiologist, Princess Royal University Hospital, Farnborough, UK

Alex N. Borg MD MRCP

Cardiology Research Registrar, Wythenshawe Hospital, Manchester, UK

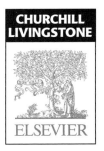

CHURCHILL
LIVINGSTONE

ELSEVIER

Edinburgh   London   New York   Oxford   Philadelphia   St Louis   Sydney   Toronto   2006

ELSEVIER
CHURCHILL
LIVINGSTONE

First published 2006

ISBN-10: 0 443 10183 3
ISBN-13: 9780 443 10183 0
IE ISBN-10: 0 443 10182 5
IE ISBN-13: 9780 443 10182 3

British Library Cataloguing in Publication Data
A catalogue record for this book is available from the British Library

Library of Congress Cataloging in Publication Data
A catalog record for this book is available from the Library of Congress

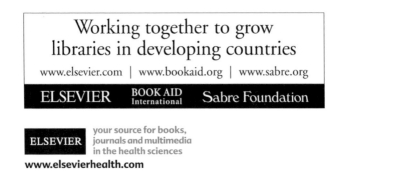

Working together to grow
libraries in developing countries

www.elsevier.com | www.bookaid.org | www.sabre.org

ELSEVIER   BOOK AID International   Sabre Foundation

ELSEVIER   your source for books, journals and multimedia in the health sciences
www.elsevierhealth.com

The publisher's policy is to use paper manufactured from sustainable forests

Printed in China

Preface

This ECG book is different.

Because electrocardiography isn't just about ECG interpretation, Chapter 1 places the subject in context and provides a historical as well as theoretical insight into the origins of the ECG. Chapter 2 is devoted entirely to the practical aspects of ECG recording drawn from many years of experience. It provides hints and tips to help you when performing an ECG and on how to identify and correct those things which might go wrong. By the end of Chapter 2 you will be well equipped to produce the perfect ECG every time. It also describes the common pitfalls associated with recording which ultimately affect interpretation.

Chapter 3 covers ECG interpretation in a straightforward way, and is designed for easy reference. All aspects of interpretation are described in a unique, easy-to-follow format that doesn't demand daring feats of memory but rather acts as a tool and guide to the correct diagnosis. All of the cardiac rhythms and abnormalities likely to be encountered in practice are included.

The uncomplicated, comprehensive treatment of the subject matter and the informal style make *ECG Complete* suitable for both the absolute beginner and the more experienced reader. It is an especially useful text for medical students in their clinical training, cardiac physiologists taking the Society for Cardiological Science and Technology exams and for student nurses. If you're new to the ECG, or are looking for a definitive reference source to carry around, this book might be for you.

Acknowledgements

We would like to acknowledge the help of Dr Stephan Brincat, Jane Webb, Martyn Bucknall and all the staff in the Clinical Measurements Department at the Princess Royal University Hospital, Farnborough, Jan Rogers, Chris Burke, Vanessa Bowbrick and Marion Borg Muscat.

S. B.
A. B.

Contents

ECG basics and history

INTRODUCTION

The first time you hold an ECG in your hands you may be troubled by a few questions.

For instance, why are the waves called P, Q, R, S, T and not A, B, C, D, E? And what do they mean? Why do P waves look round and R waves look pointed? And why do they look different in different leads? Anyway, what is a "lead" and why do we need 12 of them? You may also like to know how it's possible to detect the heart's activity from the surface of the skin and why, indeed, do we bother to record an ECG at all?

After you have read this chapter you will be able to answer all of these questions and a whole lot more besides. Perhaps you might then spare a thought for all the frog amputees and the dogs with angina who made the electrocardiogram, as we know it today, possible in the first place.

ECG ORIGINS

The first human electrocardiogram was not recorded until 1887, and then not in any quantifiable fashion until 1901. In order for this to happen a number of new discoveries had to be made, a few well-crafted experiments had to be conducted and quite a bit of luck was necessary along the way.

In 1780 Italian anatomist Luigi Galvani made a chance discovery. While working in his laboratory in the University of Bologna, Galvani noticed that upon touching the nerve in a frog's leg with a scalpel the muscle in the leg appeared to contract. Inspired, Galvani was soon attaching frogs via brass hooks to an iron rail in his garden and observing that the frog's legs twitched during lightening storms. He concluded that this was due to the presence of "animal electricity" which, he postulated, was released by the brain and flowed through the nerves to activate the muscles. Later, in 1791 Galvani went on to describe the electrical stimulation of a frog's heart leading to its contraction. The connection between electricity and the contraction of the heart was thus made.

It wasn't until almost thirty years later in 1819 that a Danish physicist called Hans Christian Oersted, whilst demonstrating to students the heating of a platinum wire with electricity, noticed a nearby compass needle moving every time the electricity was turned on. Oersted, adopted son of a German wigmaker, had inadvertently discovered the basis of electromagnetism. This discovery lead a German scientist named Johann Schweigger to postulate that a current-carrying wire produced a magnetic field. Schweigger found that if he wrapped a piece of wire many times around a coil and then passed an electric current though it the effect on the magnetised needle could be multiplied. The size of the deflection on the needle could therefore be related to the size of the electric current passing through the wire. On the 16th September 1820 Schweigger announced his new invention. He called it the galvanometer (after Galvani) and this was to become the basis of the modern day ECG machine.

For the first time scientists had an instrument capable of measuring electric current. Unfortunately, a few problems existed with the early device. Firstly, although it could detect the presence of a current, it was too insensitive to accurately measure it. Secondly, it was subject to the interference produced by the Earth's magnetic field. It was a further five years of tinkering before Italian physiologist Leopoldo Nobili developed what was called the "astatic" galvanometer. Without the external interference the galvanometer's sensitivity was greatly increased. Two years later Nobili was the first to use the instrument to directly measure electric currents in a frog.

However, despite the galvanometer's apparent promise, eighteenth century physiologists inherently distrusted the device and frogs, once again, would provide the solution.

Carlo Matteucci, professor of physics at the University of Pisa, took and perfected a method of measuring electric current previously demonstrated by Galvani. This method, delightfully called the rheoscopic frog, was a simple preparation basically consisting of a frog's leg in a jar. The cut nerve acted as an electrical sensor, the twitching of the leg as a visual representation of the presence of an electric current. Using this method Matteucci was able to demonstrate the presence of an electric current accompanying each heart beat. As primitive as such a method now might seem physiologists of the time seemed to prefer the organic basis of the rheoscopic frog to the comparatively mechanised galvanometer. However, in spite of Matteucci's success the galvanometer would make a number of important reappearances.

By 1843 German physiologist Emil Dubois-Reymond had made further improvements to the galvanometer by increasing the number of turns of wire on the coil to 24,000 (a staggering 5 km of wire in total). Using this he was able to detect a small voltage present in resting muscle tissue. This voltage was noted to change as the muscle contracted and DuBois-Reymond described his findings as an "action potential".

Later in 1856, Rudolph Von Koelliker and Heinrich Müller confirmed Matteucci's findings this time using a mechanical galvanometer. Additionally, and more significantly, they recorded the presence of a small "action potential" prior to ventricular systole.

What is an action potential?

The term action potential requires some explanation at this point because it underpins the basis of cardiac electricity at a cellular level. The heart is composed of essentially two types of cells – the myocytes (cardiac muscle cells responsible for contraction) and the specialised cells of the conduction system (see below). An action potential is the point at which the cells become electrically activated and, in the case of cardiac myocytes, contract. What we know now is that the flow of ions (electrically charged particles) in and out of the cells sets up an electric potential across the cell membrane and the cells, when they are resting, are said to be *polarised*.

This is analogous to the muscle tissues studied by Dubois-Reymond. The resting membrane potential of the atrial and ventricular myocytes is said to be stable until external excitation occurs. Excitation is initiated via the specialised conduction system because the cells of the conduction system are said to be "unstable".

To consider this a bit further let's take an example. We know that the heart's normal rhythm, sinus rhythm, is produced, as its name implies, by the sinus node. The sinus node is formed by a small strip of modified muscle cells which lie on the posterior wall of the right atrium at the junction with the superior vena cava (Fig. 1.1). The sinus node

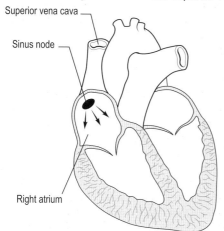

Superior vena cava

Sinus node

Right atrium

◀ **Fig. 1.1** Position of sinus node in right atrium.

3

is the first part of the heart's specialised conduction system and it is from here that the heart's normal rhythm is initiated.

The cells of the sinus node possess a special characteristic called self-excitability. As such they are able to spontaneously depolarise via electrochemical gradients which exist across their very permeable cell membranes. If you were to place a microelectrode within the cell you would find, just as Du Bois-Reymond did, that there is a voltage present in the resting cell in the region of minus 60mV. As an increasing amount of positive sodium ions enter from outside of the cell the voltage becomes increasingly positive and the cell begins to depolarise. Once the voltage reaches a critical value (at around minus 40 mV) it is triggered to produce an action potential. An action potential results in the "firing" of the sinus node. The sinus node depolarises on average just over once every second causing the heart to beat at a rate of between 60 and 70 times every minute. The cells then return to their resting state via a process of *repolarisation*. During this time positively-charged potassium ions are actively being pumped out of the cell. Hence the inside of the cell becomes *less positive* and the resting state is restored.

Up until the invention of the mercury capillary electrometer by Gabriel Lippmann in 1872 it was necessary to open the chest of the subject to expose the heart so that measurements of cardiac electricity could be made. The electrometer was quite different from the galvanometer and was, at the time, considered to be a more sensitive instrument. It consisted of a glass column containing a mercury–sulfuric acid interface. Each end of the column was attached to a wire that could measure the difference in electric potential between the two ends of the tube. If a fall or rise in potential occurred at either end the meniscus would move and a measurement could be recorded. Augustus Desiré Waller was the first to attempt to record the heart's electricity using the electrometer non-invasively *and* on a human. A euphoric frog population breathed a collective sigh of relief.

Waller studied medicine in Aberdeen and Edinburgh but following qualification he moved down to London where he worked, initially, at the University College of London alongside Sir John Burdon Sanderson. Sanderson and fellow physiologist Frederick Page, were already putting the capillary electrometer to good use by recording the heart's electrical activity firstly in 1878 in a frog (showing that it consisted of two "phases") and then in a tortoise (the recordings from which were subsequently published) in 1884.

Later in the same year, Waller was appointed lecturer in physiology at St Mary's Medical School and it was here, in 1887, that he endeavoured to record the first ever human "electrogram" (as he liked to call it).

The immediate problem Waller faced was that the electrical activity of the heart is measured in the region of around 1 mV. This voltage is so small that even when the chest was opened and the heart exposed, a microscope was still necessary in order to observe the changes within the electrometer. However, his solution was the stuff of schoolboy invention. Waller shone a light through the glass column of the electrometer so that the movement of the meniscus was projected and enlarged. The light was directed at a photographic plate and the plate was moved through the light on a toy wagon pulled along by a weight. What Waller was effectively doing was recording changes in potential (as measured by the moving meniscus) against time. The ECG as we view it today, although a touch more sophisticated, essentially does just the same.

How can we detect the heart's activity from the surface of the skin?

Waller managed to generate these recordings by immersing his hands and feet in metal bowls of salty water which acted as electrodes. Waller didn't know at the time – he imagined the limbs to act as some sort of extension cables – but this is possible because the spread of electricity through the heart involves the flow of small currents through the extracellular fluid. This extracellular fluid surrounds the cells of the heart and acts as a continuous conducting medium between the heart and the skin. Hence small potential differences are detectable on the body surface – so long as you're using an appropriate electrode. Since 1887 huge advancements in electronics and electrode technology means that, thankfully, buckets of salty water are no longer necessary.

Initially Waller tried this system on himself, and later on a laboratory assistant named Thomas Goswell. Spurred on by his success he continued his experiments, changing the combinations of limbs placed in the water and even, at one point, putting a spoon in his mouth to see if he could discern a difference. Initially no difference was seen. Then, when he tried submersing his right foot and left hand he was unable to generate any observable potential at all. The result was the same when he tried both feet together. After a bit of thought Waller concluded that the direction of electricity through the body must be related to the position of the heart in the chest. Electrically speaking, the body must consist of two sides, he thought, represented as the right arm and head on one side and the rest of the body on the other. Waller postulated that the spread of electricity had its origin at the ventricular apex and ran upwards towards the atria. We now know, in fact, the reverse is true.

Orientation of the heart in the chest

The heart is approximately the size of a clenched fist and is situated in the thorax between the lungs, immediately behind the sternum (Fig. 1.2). About two-thirds of its mass lies to the left of the midline of the body with its apex (pointed end) directed roughly towards the fifth intercostal space at around the anterior axillary line (approximately in the region of your left nipple). The heart is slightly twisted in fact with the right ventricle at the top and front and the left ventricle underneath. The atria are situated above the ventricles and it is from here that the cardiac impulse arises. The direction of spread of electricity then is from top (atria) to bottom (ventricular apex) – Figure 1.3.

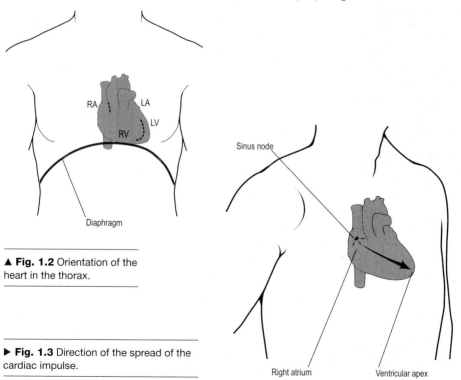

▲ **Fig. 1.2** Orientation of the heart in the thorax.

▶ **Fig. 1.3** Direction of the spread of the cardiac impulse.

5

When he wasn't experimenting on himself Waller would, like many scientists of his day, enlist the help of those around him. Waller would often arrive at public meetings in his motor car, cigar in hand and Jimmy (his trusty bulldog) at his side. The dog, of course, was always the unassuming participant in Waller's demonstrations, standing, as was necessary, with his paws in bowls of saline. It was during one such demonstration in 1889 at the First International Congress of Physiologists that a young physiologist from the Netherlands named Willem Einthoven first saw Waller performing his technique.

Einthoven was born in Semarang in the Dutch East Indies in 1860 where his father, a former army medical officer, was working as a parish doctor. After his father died in 1886 Einthoven returned with his mother and his brothers and sisters to Utrecht in Holland. It was at the University of Utrecht where Einthoven, in 1878, began his medical training, fully intending to follow in his father's footsteps. Einthoven qualified as a general practitioner in 1886, but not before being appointed Professor of Physiology at the University of Leiden. It was here that he began working with the capillary electrometer but, dissatisfied with the inertia of the instrument, he devised methods of increasing both its stability and accuracy.

Three years after Waller's demonstration two physiologists from University College, London named William Bayliss and Edward Starling were using the electrometer in their research on the electrical activity of the heart. With the use of more powerful projecting microscopes Bayliss and Starling were able to discern three separate deflections in their electrograms (Waller had identified only two). In 1895, in his first paper on the subject, Einthoven described not three but five deflections generated by his "enhanced electrometer". He labelled these deflections P, Q, R, S and T. With much of the alphabet already plundered by mathematicians for algebra the use of these letters was not just something Einthoven assigned arbitrarily – his use of these letters can be traced back to 17th century scientist René Descartes. Einthoven later discovered a sixth wave. Naturally he called it a U wave.

What do the waves mean?
And so it is that the ECG is composed of six waves (Fig. 1.4). Three of these waves form a complex. And between these waves there are two intervals and one segment.

Note that the term *isoelectric* in Table 1.1 (below) refers to the time during which the electrical charges through the heart are equal. During this time no deflection occurs on the ECG.

Why do P waves look round?
The impulse generated by the cells of the sinus node spreads across both of the atria, and is conducted cell-to-cell via special pathways called intercalated discs and protoplasmic bridges at a speed of approximately 1 metre per second (Fig. 1.5). Because atrial conduction is by a cell-to-cell method it is slower than for other parts of the conduction system and therefore the spread of depolarisation is also slower. The result is a rounded deflection on the ECG trace known as the P wave. Note that atrial repolarisation is not seen on the surface ECG because it coincides with the onset of ventricular depolarisation and is therefore hidden within the QRS complex.

The role of the atrioventricular node
The impulse is prevented from passing directly into the ventricles by the atrioventricular ring – a ring of non-conducting fibrous tissue separating the upper and lower chambers of the heart. The only way the impulse can travel, in the absence of an abnormal accessory pathway, is via the atrioventricular, or AV node.

The AV node is situated in the lower portion of the atrial septum, the wall dividing the two atria, and it has three main tasks.

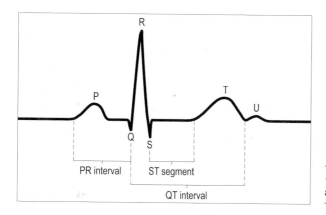

◀ **Fig. 1.4** ECG waveforms and intervals.

Table 1.1: What do the waves mean?

Deflection	What it represents
P wave	Atrial depolarisation
PR interval	Time delay between atrial depolarisation and ventricular activation
QRS complex	Ventricular depolarisation
ST segment (isoelectric)	Electrical plateau of ventricular activation
T wave	Ventricular repolarisation
QT interval	Total time for ventricular depolarisation and repolarisation
U wave	Possibly septal or late ventricular repolarisation

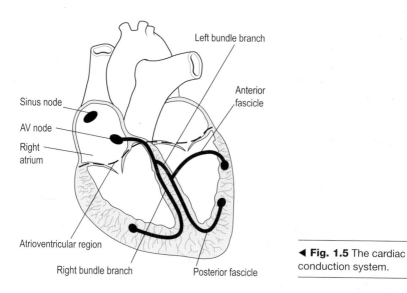

◀ **Fig. 1.5** The cardiac conduction system.

Firstly it acts to delay the impulse. Conduction through the AV node is at a speed of 0.2 metres per second. This slower speed allows time for the ventricles to fill with blood so that the optimum amount of blood can be passed from atria to ventricles to be pumped around the body. This delay in conduction accounts for the PR interval.

Secondly, the AV node acts as a secondary pacemaker. This is known as *automaticity* and the AV node can produce heart rates of between 45–60 bpm. This is particularly important if one part of the conduction system fails. For instance, if the sinus node fails to fire, the AV node may take over and set the rate of the heart beat.

Thirdly, the AV node acts like a kind of electrical filter so that if the atria begin to fire off impulses at unusually high rates it is the job of the AV node to "block" the extra impulses and prevent them from being transmitted through to the ventricles and causing dangerously fast heart rates.

Why are R waves pointed?

The bundle of His and the bundle branches

The conducting tissue connecting the atria to the ventricles was discovered by His in 1892. The His bundle is made up of fast conducting tissue and occupies the fibrous part of the upper interventricular septum, the wall dividing the two ventricles. From here the bundle divides into the left bundle branch which supplies the left ventricle and the right bundle branch supplying the right ventricle. The left bundle is really made up of two distinct fibres, called fascicles, supplying the anterior and posterior portions of the left ventricle respectively.

Purkinje fibres

Named after the Hungarian histologist who first described them in 1845, the Purkinje fibres emerge from the terminals of the bundle branches and form a vast branching network which travel deep into the surrounding heart muscle. The speed of conduction through the Purkinje fibres is in the region of between 3–5 metres per second and is thus very fast.

The cells of both the His bundle and the Purkinje fibres also demonstrate automaticity and are able to act, like the AV node, as subsidiary pacemakers. The bundle of His is able to spontaneously depolarise at a rate of around 40 bpm. The Purkinje fibres produce rates between 15–30 bpm.

Because depolarisation of the ventricles is via fast conducting fibres and the ventricular muscle mass is greater than in the atria, the impulse travels much faster and produces a higher voltage. This results in a sharp, pointed deflection on the ECG trace known as the R wave. Depending on which lead you look at on an ECG, and also because the interventricular septum depolarises in an overall left to right direction, there may also be associated Q waves and S waves. The components of the QRS complex are defined as follows:

- Q wave – the first negative (downward) deflection following the P wave
- R Wave – the first positive (upward) deflection following the P wave whether or not it is preceded by a Q wave
- S wave – the first negative deflection following an R wave.

The QRS complex so formed coincides with the contraction of the ventricles and ventricular systole.

The ST segment

The ventricle during this phase of the ECG is uniformly depolarised. Hence the ST segment is usually isoelectric.

T waves

T waves represent ventricular *repolarisation*. This is the time during which the cells in the ventricles are recovering from their influx of positive ions and are returning to their polarised resting states.

The QT interval

This is the total time taken for the ventricles to depolarise and then repolarise and is dependent on the prevailing heart rate.

The U wave

U waves are rather elusive and aren't present on all ECGs. Even when they are present they are not always easily seen (or may otherwise be mistaken for extra P waves). It is thought that they may represent either septal repolarisation or delayed ventricular repolarisation. Either way, nobody seems to know for certain.

Einthoven's awareness of further improvements to the galvanometer by French physicist Arene D'Arsonval and French engineer Clement Ader lead him to return to his pursuit of more sensitive measuring devices and in 1901 he announced his modifications to the string galvanometer (as it was now known). While acknowledging the work of D'Arsonval and Ader, Einthoven did what any self-respecting physiologist should do and pointed out that his galvanometer was much better (it was in fact many thousands of times more sensitive than their's). What Einthoven additionally achieved was the introduction of a standardised technique for recording which is still used today. Einthoven's photographic plate was calibrated to move at a rate of 25 mm each second so that each 1 mm deflection represented 0.04 seconds.

Einthoven's work was, at the same time, becoming more clinical. He noted that each patient had his own characteristic electrocardiogram (as Einthoven preferred to call it) but observed that all of these essentially conformed to a general type. From this basic understanding he was able to go on to show that different forms of heart disease manifest themselves in particular ways. In 1903 he recorded and described electrocardiograms in atrial enlargement, atrial fibrillation, atrial flutter, ventricular premature contractions (along with ventricular bigeminy) and heart block experimentally induced in a dog.

Einthoven's triangle and the concept of a lead

From Waller's work, Einthoven knew that the appearance of the ECG depended on where on the body the measuring electrodes were placed. As Waller had observed, the combination of certain sites resulted in no measured potential at all. Einthoven proposed a standardised three lead system measured from specific points on the body. For improved accuracy Einthoven recommended these three leads be recorded simultaneously. Note that one "lead" is formed from the combination of two or more measuring electrodes. Because we are dealing with electricity here, each lead has a positive and a negative end (pole) and leads I, II and III (as Einthoven called them) are therefore termed *bipolar* leads. Bipolar leads represent a difference of electric potential between two selected electrode sites. By placing electrodes on each of the limbs Einthoven said that lead I records the difference in potential between the right arm and left arm, lead II the difference between the right arm and the left leg, and lead III the difference between the left arm and the left leg.

$$\text{Lead I} = \text{LA}(+) + \text{RA}(-)$$
$$\text{Lead II} = \text{LL}(+) + \text{RA}(-)$$
$$\text{Lead III} = \text{LL}(+) + \text{LA}(-)$$

Einthoven expressed the relationship between these three leads as:

$$\text{Lead III} = \text{Lead II} - \text{Lead I}$$

This means that the degree of potential difference recorded in lead III is equal to the difference in potential (recorded simultaneously) between leads I and II.

In 1912 Einthoven addressed the Chelsea Clinical Society in London and described an equilateral triangle formed by his three leads. This was later referred to as "Einthoven's triangle". The theory behind Einthoven's triangle states that the heart is at the centre of an equilateral triangle with apices at the left arm, the right arm and the left leg (Fig. 1.6).

Einthoven was unquestionably one of the most important figures in early electro-cardiography and was recognised as such in 1924 when he was awarded the Nobel prize in Physiology or Medicine for his work.

Wilson's central terminal

In 1931 Frank Wilson of the University of Michigan in the United States first described the concept of a unipolar lead system which utilised what he called an "exploring elec-trode". This electrode could be used to record the activity of the heart from anywhere on the body. Wilson later introduced three additional leads formed from the average potential measured between any two of Einthoven's standard leads. These were:

> Lead VR = right arm paired with the average of the left arm and left foot
> Lead VL = left arm paired with the average of the left foot and right arm
> Lead VF = left foot paired with the average of the left and right arms.

This can perhaps be seen more clearly from the diagram below. Note that the abbre-viations stand for voltage, right, left and foot respectively. To achieve these additional leads required a clever bit of electronics and Wilson incorporated 5000 ohm resistors to each electrode terminal which, when combined, formed what was to be called "Wilson's central terminal". Because of the electrical configuration of these leads they are often referred to as unipolar leads (Fig. 1.7).

Goldberger's augmented leads

The voltage acquired from Wilson's three leads was initially very small. With a little bit more electronic dabbling Emmanuel Goldberger, in 1942, was able to increase the de-rived voltages by 50%. A slight change of name was in order and the leads then became known as aVR, aVL and aVF (where "a" means augmented).

Because leads I, II, III and aVR, aVL and aVF are all acquired by placing electrodes on the limbs, they are often referred to collectively as the "limb leads".

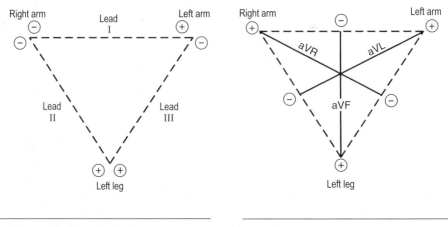

▲ **Fig. 1.6** Einthoven's triangle.

▲ **Fig. 1.7** The unipolar limb leads incorporated into Einthoven's triangle.

The precordial (chest) leads

The development of Wilson's central terminal and the "exploring electrode" allowed the introduction of six additional unipolar leads recorded from across the precordium (the front of the chest). In 1938 the American Heart Association and the Cardiac Society of Great Britain defined the standard positions of these chest leads and respectively labelled them V1–V6.

So why do we need 12 leads?

A quick bit of mental arithmetic at this point and you should see that we now have 12 leads in total: three standard bipolar limb leads courtesy of Einthoven, three unipolar augmented leads care of Wilson and Goldberger plus an additional six chest leads into the bargain. But why have 12 leads at all? Why not have fewer leads (since three leads seemed to work so well for Einthoven)?

The value of the ECG in routine use is optimal with 12 leads. Recording fewer leads may be acceptable when simply monitoring the cardiac rhythm but is detrimental to the reliability of the ECG in other situations. Having 12 leads affords us the opportunity to view the heart from a number of perspectives. Without the precordial leads it would become difficult – if not impossible – to detect abnormalities such as anterior or posterior myocardial infarction and differentiate left and right bundle branch block. Also, lead V1 often allows us best visualisation of P waves. Additionally, the limb leads enable us to determine the cardiac axis and allow us to determine the presence of inferior myocardial infarction.

On the other hand, it is acceptable – and indeed desirable – to include additional leads particularly in the case of infants, patients with dextrocardia or in the detection of right ventricular and posterior myocardial infarction. But recording more leads routinely has produced varying degrees of success and does not appear to add much to the overall sensitivity and specificity of the test outside of these particular circumstances.

Until studies into coronary occlusion were published in the early 1900s there was still some debate and general bickering about why we might bother to record an ECG in the first place. Waller had regarded the ECG more as a physiologist's aid to understanding the heart's electricity rather than a clinical tool in itself. No such doubts existed in the mind of Einthoven who, meanwhile, was busy recording ECGs in his Leiden laboratory via telephone lines from patients in a nearby hospital. Recognising the clinical potential of the ECG machine he discussed its possible manufacture with the Cambridge Scientific Instrument Company in London. While Einthoven was certain of its usefulness, critics pointed out that the ECG did not change the way patients were managed (in fact quinidine and digitalis therapy remained the standard treatment for most of the cardiac arrhythmias described by Einthoven until the 1950s).

The ECG as a clinical tool became more important as physicians began to recognise acute coronary syndromes. In 1912, American physician James B. Herrick reported the clinical and pathological features of sudden coronary artery occlusion. However, the medical community didn't begin to reevaluate the usefulness of the ECG until 1918, when a paper published by Dr Fred Smith – Herrick's assistant – described typical ECG patterns associated with artificially-induced myocardial infarction in dogs. Smith opened the chests of sixty dogs, tied off one of the coronary arteries "with strong linen", closed the chests and then recorded serial ECGs over the ensuing hours and days. What Smith observed was a pattern of changes that were dependent on which artery had been ligated. Additionally Smith found that these changes were frequently accompanied by increasing numbers of premature ventricular contractions sometimes leading to tachycardia (rapid heart rates) or even fibrillation (rapid disorganised contractions).

Smith's study was unfortunately dogged (no pun intended) by his use of only three

ECG leads (leads I, II and III). It was to be another 13 years before Wilson would introduce the concept of unipolar leads and another 20 years before the standard positions of the precordial leads would be defined. Regardless, from Smith's results Herrick was able to conjecture at the possibility of being able to determine the site of infarction from a particular pattern on a patient's ECG. Subsequent pathological studies supported this view. In the few years following Smith's investigation it became accepted that diagnostic ECG changes were associated with the clinical syndrome of acute myocardial infarction, the term "injury current" was introduced to describe ST segment elevation and it became generally accepted that ST segment elevation occurring in particular ECG leads represented the underlying area of myocardium and site of occlusion.

WHICH LEADS LOOK AT WHICH SURFACES OF THE HEART?

These days the surfaces of the heart, for the purposes of ECG interpretation, are defined as follows:

- the anterior surface (the top) made up largely by the right ventricle
- the posterior surface (the back) made up almost completely by the left atrium
- the inferior surface (the bottom) consisting mostly of the left ventricle with a small area of right ventricle
- the lateral surface (the side) made up by the edge of the left ventricle (Fig. 1.8).

There are two main coronary arteries supplying all of these surfaces and these are named simply, the right coronary artery (RCA) and the left coronary artery (LCA). Both arteries originate from the aorta just above the aortic valve.

The right coronary artery, in the majority of patients, supplies largely the inferior and posterior surfaces of the heart. The left coronary artery supplies both the anterior and lateral surfaces in the majority of patients and branches from its main stem into two sections: the left anterior descending artery (LAD) and the circumflex artery (supplying the lateral aspect).

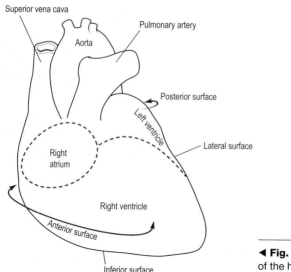

◄ **Fig. 1.8** The surfaces of the heart.

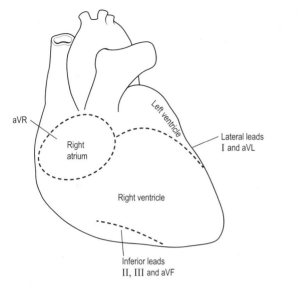

Table 1.2: Surfaces of the heart – the limb leads

Lead	Surface of the heart
I	Lateral
II	Inferior
III	Inferior
aVR	Right atrial territory
aVL	High lateral
aVF	Inferior

◀ **Fig. 1.9** Lead view points (limb leads).

Understanding which leads of the ECG look at which surfaces of the heart, and by extension, which coronary artery supplies a particular territory becomes important in the diagnosis of acute myocardial infarction where, as we have seen, there is a good correlation between ECG changes in a particular lead and the underlying coronary occlusion.

The limb leads I, II, III, aVR, aVL and aVF look at the heart in the frontal (or coronal) plane (Fig. 1.9). The areas of the heart viewed by each lead are shown in Table 1.2 above.

The precordial (or chest) leads have specific anatomical positions across the chest and these look at the heart in the horizontal (or transverse) plane (Fig. 1.10).

The surfaces of the heart viewed by each chest lead are shown in Table 1.3.

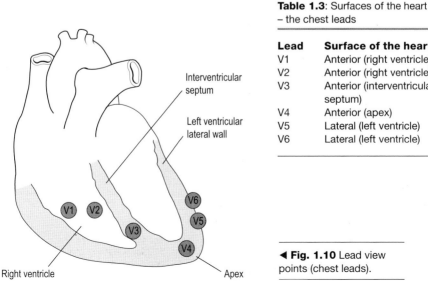

Table 1.3: Surfaces of the heart – the chest leads

Lead	Surface of the heart
V1	Anterior (right ventricle)
V2	Anterior (right ventricle)
V3	Anterior (interventricular septum)
V4	Anterior (apex)
V5	Lateral (left ventricle)
V6	Lateral (left ventricle)

◀ **Fig. 1.10** Lead view points (chest leads).

WHY DOES THE ECG LOOK DIFFERENT IN DIFFERENT LEADS?

As already stated, the spread of depolarisation of the heart is in a general south-easterly direction from top to bottom. Because the wave of depolarisation has both magnitude and direction it is called a *vector*. From first principles, if our vector is travelling toward a lead then we will get a positive deflection on our ECG. If on the other hand the vector is travelling away from a particular lead, we will get a negative deflection. If the vector is travelling perpendicular to a lead we will see a complex that is *equiphasic*. This means that the deflection on our ECG will be neither predominantly positive nor negative but somewhere in between.

Patterns in the chest leads

Depolarisation spreads to the ventricles via the interventricular septum. The septum depolarises with an initial left-to-right vector. This will produce a small Q wave in the left-sided chest leads (V5 & V6) as depolarisation is initially travelling away from these leads. For the right-sided chest leads (V1 & V2) this will produce a small R wave (Fig. 1.11).

As the depolarisation spreads through the bundle branches across the ventricular muscle a large R wave will result in the left-sided leads. The deflection is positive because the depolarisation vector is toward the electrodes and large because the left ventricle has such a large muscle mass. Deep S waves will occur in the right-sided leads due to this extra mass as the greater part of the depolarisation vector is travelling away from them.

The overall result is an rS complex in V1 and a qR complex in V6. The size of the letters here relates to the size of the respective vectors as depicted by each lead.

Lead V3, in many patients, is oriented toward the septum and so tends to be equiphasic, meaning that the complex is as much positive as it is negative. This is called the *transition zone* because from this point onwards the ECG complexes change from being predominantly negative to becoming predominantly positive.

Patterns in the limb leads: the mean frontal plane QRS axis

As we have seen, the limb leads look at the heart in what is called the frontal plane.

Remember that the six limb leads are formed from Einthoven's three standard leads (forming Einthoven's Triangle) and from the three Wilson/Goldberger augmented unipolar leads.

Einthoven's triangle can be geometrically deconstructed to form a reference system,

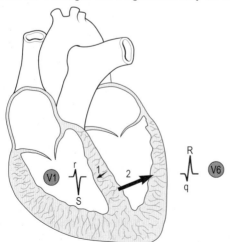

◀ **Fig. 1.11** Pattern of depolarisation in the chest leads.

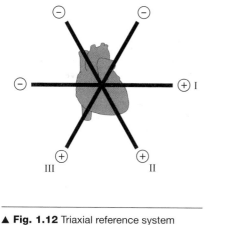

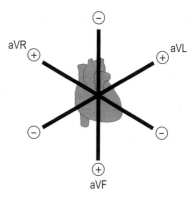

▲ **Fig. 1.12** Triaxial reference system (bipolar leads).

▲ **Fig. 1.13** Triaxial reference system (unipolar leads).

which, because it is composed of three axes, is called a *triaxial* reference system, as shown in Figure 1.12 above.

As can be seen, each lead is separated by 60 degrees. With the heart at the centre of such a system it is easier to see how lead I looks at the lateral surface of the heart and leads II and III at the inferior surface. As you can see lead II looks at the heart from the bottom up. Depolarisation is travelling toward the ventricles from the atria and so toward lead II. The result is a complex with positive P, R and T waves.

The three unipolar limb leads can also be geometrically deconstructed into a triaxial reference system (Fig. 1.13). As you can see, aVR looks at the heart from the approximate direction of the right atrium. In this lead the wave of depolarisation produced from the sinus node is travelling away from the right atrium towards the ventricles. The resulting complex therefore appears inverted with negative (or upside down) P, R and T waves. aVL forms a further lateral lead, and aVF is the third inferior lead.

SO WHAT CAN AN ECG TELL US?

The ECG is one of the most requested routine tests in medicine and is a fundamental tool in cardiology. It is perhaps most useful in the detection and identification of cardiac arrhythmias where it is still considered to be the gold standard. It is also a principal part in the diagnosis and treatment of myocardial infarction and other forms of heart disease. You should be aware, however, that there are fewer recognisable ECG patterns than there are potential pathophysiologies. Moreover, it is possible for two or more pathophysiologies to coexist and so the sensitivity and specificity of the ECG in these circumstances is further reduced. It is important to stress, therefore, that an ECG should be used as an aid to diagnosis and should never be considered in isolation.

Nevertheless, the ECG forms a requisite part of monitoring in coronary and intensive care units, in the cardiac catheterisation laboratory, and during surgical intervention (where it also acts as an important aid during the pre- and postoperative phases) and is increasingly becoming a feature in GP surgeries. It has many practical applications, particularly in 24 hour Holter monitoring and in combination with a treadmill or other types of exercise testing. Additionally, it may also play an important role in diseases of the pulmonary system, during electrolyte disturbances, in renal disease and in the detection of abnormalities secondary to certain types of drugs. Appropriate evaluation of cardiac pacemakers would be virtually impossible without the aid of an ECG.

Einthoven's ECG machine weighed a massive 600 pounds and was thus stuck in his Leiden laboratory. ECG machines these days are portable, easy to use, non-invasive, and relatively inexpensive.

The reliability of the ECG is dependent to a great extent on the quality and accuracy of the data recorded and it is therefore important that you should be competent in the practical aspects of recording. This forms the subject of the next chapter.

Glossary of some important terms

- **Polarised** – the "resting" electrical state of a cell

- **Depolarised/depolarisation** – the change in electrical state of a cell due to the inflow of positively-charged ions.

- **Action potential** – the point at which a cell becomes electrically activated

- **Isoelectric** – the time during which the electrical charges through the heart are equal. During this time no deflection occurs on the ECG

- **Automaticity** – the property of a cell which allows it to spontaneously depolarise

- **Repolarisation** – the process of a return to the normal resting state of a cell following an action potential

- **ECG lead** – formed from the combination of two or more electrodes

- **Einthoven's triangle** – a theoretical triangle describing the electrical aspects of the bipolar limb leads

- **Bipolar** – literally meaning "two poles". Electrically speaking, a positive and a negative end

- **Triaxial reference system** – theoretical system composed of three axes describing the electrical reference points of the ECG limb leads

- **Equiphasic** – meaning "equal phase". The positive component of the ECG is equal to the negative component

- **Transition zone** – the point at which an equiphasic complex is produced in the chest leads indicating both the position of the septum and a change in the precordial leads to predominantly positive complexes (usually occurring around lead V3)

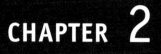
The ECG in practice

INTRODUCTION

The process of producing an accurate, good quality ECG is quite straightforward providing you develop a good technique. A poor quality trace not only reduces the accuracy of the test but also makes interpretation difficult and sometimes impossible. Even if your job does not involve ECG recording you should still be aware of the points made in the following pages. Failure to recognise interference, unmarked changes in standard calibration settings or incorrect electrode placement can all lead to erroneous diagnosis and unnecessary treatment or interventions. If your job does involve ECG recording it is important that you are able to record an ECG from different types of patients in different circumstances. Further, you should be able to adapt your technique to different clinical settings. For instance, which leads would you additionally record for a patient with dextrocardia or suspected posterior myocardial infarction? Some patients are excessively hairy, some are infectious. Some are missing limbs and others may be incapable of lying on a couch. What do you do then?

This chapter describes the practical aspects of ECG recording and also includes sub-sections on ambulatory monitoring and the ECG exercise test (two practical applications).

HOW TO RECORD AN ECG

Patient approach
The ECG is far easier to perform if the patient is well-informed about the procedure, made comfortable and put at ease. All top items of clothing should be removed along with tights or long boots. The patient should be asked to lie down and made comfortable by adjusting the position of the bed and adding or removing pillows as required. Arms should be resting loosely by their sides.

Skin preparation
Because the quality of the signal you will record depends largely on the skin–electrode interface you are able to generate, skin abrasion is fundamental to the procedure. Abrasion not only helps to clean the skin at the electrode site but also helps to reduce skin impedance. Skin impedance exists in a range between 1 Kohm (in the case of normal skin) to around 1000 Kohms (in the case of dry skin) and acts to attenuate the size of the signal measurable by the ECG machine. The use of a paper towel or tissue during abrading is usually all that is needed – it is often quite adequate to give the patient just a quick rub at each electrode site. Excessive rubbing has not been shown to reduce skin impedance much further and the use of abrasive pads should be reserved only for those patients in whom it is difficult to obtain a good quality trace.

Some practitioners use alcohol swabs to clean the skin surface before applying electrodes. Alcohol dries out the skin and adds to the skin impedance if not properly wiped away before application. Hence any use of alcohol should be followed by abrasion with a dry paper towel or tissue.

There is occasionally some argument about whether a patient's chest should be shaved for an ECG. Hair is a non-conductive material that not only prevents good electrical contact but also compromises electrode adhesion. However, there is an infection risk associated with shaving. If the hair can be easily parted and a good contact made with the electrode then shaving the chest should not be necessary. Still, there are a few men in whom the chest hair is too dense to part. As a general rule of thumb if *not* shaving the chest will compromise the validity of the test then shaving, with the patient's consent, is the only alternative.

To summarise then, before applying electrodes:

Abrade skin at electrode site until pink using a paper towel or wet tissue and then dry

Or
(for patients wearing creams/moisturisers such as dermatology patients)
Clean area with alcohol wipe or soapy tissue
Dry skin at site and abrade until pink

Or
(for hairy patients)
Shave away hair from electrode site (if hair cannot be parted)
Clear away loose hairs
Clean with alcohol wipe or soapy tissue and dry.

Different people use different methods, but as long as the skin is cleaned and abraded and the resulting trace is free from artifacts the method is not quite as important as the result.

ECG electrodes

Electrodes used for patient monitoring have two important functions. Firstly they allow adequate adhesion to the skin surface and, secondly, they convert the small ionic signals from the skin into an electrical current which can be seen, via a lead wire, on an ECG machine. Typically these electrodes are composed of either an aqueous conducting gel mounted on a sticky pad or a silver/silver-chloride combination which forms a part of a smaller sticky tab. Either may be connected to an ECG lead by means of a press stud or modified crocodile clip. When applying the aqueous gel-type electrodes it is important to only push on the adhesive area (often running a finger around the circumference of the electrode) as pressing on the area containing the gel may cause the gel to leak, reducing adhesion.

Electrodes come in many different shapes and sizes and are suited to different environments and patients. Because different electrodes introduce variable levels of impedance into the ECG circuit it is advised that electrodes of different construction should not be mixed on the same patient as this might result in significant variations in the amplitude of the measured signals.

Electrode positioning

For the standard 12 lead ECG you will require 10 electrodes per patient. You will remember from the previous chapter that one "lead" is produced from the placement of two or more electrodes so that all of the ECG leads you will record are formed as shown in Table 2.1.

Table 2.1 ECG leads derived from standard electrode positions

Electrode position	ECG lead produced
LA + RA	I
LL + RA	II
LL + LA	III
(LA + LL) + RA	aVR
(RA + LL) + LA	aVL
(RA + LA) + LL	aVF
(LA + RA + LL) + V	V1–V6

Where LA = left arm, RA = right arm, LL = left leg and V = any chest lead

Remember that the augmented unipolar leads (VR, VL and VF) are formed from the average potential measured between any two of standard leads (I, II and III). As you can see from the table this is a similar situation for the chest leads. This is why you can record twelve "leads" on your ECG but have only 10 cables on your ECG machine. Note that the right leg electrode is used by the ECG machine as a ground and as such plays no part in the formation of any lead.

Positioning of the limb electrodes

Limb leads should ideally be placed on the wrists and ankles but for best practice may be applied anywhere on the arms and legs as long as they are at least 15 cm away from the heart. Any less than 15 cm may affect the cardiac axis. It is advised that for a resting ECG, arm electrodes are never placed on the clavicles and leg electrodes never placed on the trunk. The right leg electrode can, however, be placed anywhere on the body but is positioned on the right leg for convenience.

Hints and Tips

- Orientate the limb electrodes with tab ends (where the electrodes are connected to the leads) pointing in the direction of the bed so that once the leads are attached they are not peeled away from the skin.
- It is recommended that you place the limb electrodes first because in a time-sensitive situation, once connected to the ECG machine, this will at least provide you with an immediate rhythm strip. The chest leads can then be placed afterwards.

Positioning of the chest electrodes

Care should be taken in determining the correct positioning of the chest electrodes because they look at particular regions of the heart from specific locations. Accurate location of these electrodes will require a great deal of fingering of the patient's chest so you should be familiar with the anatomy of the rib cage and, in particular, the sternum (Fig. 2.1).

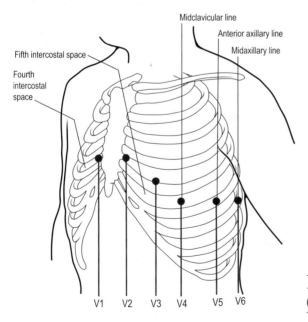

Midclavicular line
Anterior axillary line
Midaxillary line
Fifth intercostal space
Fourth intercostal space

V1 V2 V3 V4 V5 V6

◀ **Fig. 2.1** Electrode positions (chest leads).

The sternum is the flat narrow bone located in the centre of the chest and is roughly 15 cm in total length. It is composed of three basic parts, namely the manubrium (upper portion, with the suprasternal notch at its most superior point), the body (the middle, largest portion) and the xiphoid process (the lowest and smallest portion). The manubrium articulates with the first and second ribs and forms a junction with the body of the sternum at the sternal angle (or angle of Louis).

It is the sternal angle that should provide the starting point for your electrode placement. Firstly, slide a finger over the manubrium until the sternal angle is felt. Moving your finger just below this and to the left or the right locates the second intercostal space. Note that the second intercostal space should be felt just below the second rib. From this position slide your finger down to the fourth intercostal space, counting the third space on the way. This is the position, on either side of the main sternal body, for your V1 and V2 electrodes. It is perhaps best to locate the V1 and V2 positions separately rather than attempt to line up the V2 electrode adjacent to the V1 position because in some patients the ribs do not provide such convenient symmetry. Note that you are placing your electrodes in the intercostal spaces and not on the ribs themselves.

Hints and Tips

- Take care! If your electrodes in the V1 and V2 positions are placed too high on the chest (i.e. if you manage to miscount) this will electrocardiographically mimic an old septal myocardial infarction.
- Note that if your placements of V1 and V2 are incorrect and this is your starting position, all of your other leads will also be incorrectly placed. It is therefore imperative that you get this right. Some practitioners recommend using the first rib as the anatomical starting point. However, the first rib is often obscured by the clavicle and it is not always apparent that this is the case. This process is therefore prone to error.

From the fourth intercostal space slide your finger away from the sternum and count down to the fifth intercostal space. It is necessary to move away from the sternum at this point because the lower ribs fuse around the base of the sternal body and you may not be able to feel the intercostal spaces accurately around the sternal edge. The V4 electrode should be positioned in the fifth intercostal space in the midclavicular line. This position can be determined by locating the mid-point of the clavicle (where the clavicle bows) and tracing it down to the fifth intercostal space either with a finger or visually. You should always place the V4 electrode before the V3 electrode because V3 is a position midway (or equidistant) between V2 and V4.

Hints and Tips

- The fifth intercostal space in the midclavicular line is particularly difficult to find in obese patients or in patients with large breasts. It is often the case that the intercostal space cannot be felt because it falls beneath the breast tissue. In these circumstances it is worth attempting to feel the fifth intercostal space from below the breast although this is not always possible either. You should however always endeavour to place the electrode as close as is possible to the correct position and preferably not on the breast itself. Placing an electrode on top of the breast, further away from the chest wall, results in a degree of attenuation of the measured signal.

Placement of the V5 and V6 electrodes should now be straightforward. The V5 electrode is positioned horizontal to V4 in the anterior axillary line. If the patient's left arm is resting at their side, the anterior axillary line is found from the crease of skin formed between the arm and the chest (around the region of the armpit). The V6 electrode is then placed on the same horizontal line as the V5 electrode in the midaxillary line (a point from the centre of the armpit).

> **Hints and Tips**
> ● Rotate the electrodes in the V5 and V6 positions so that the tab ends are pointing down towards the bed. This is so that once the leads are attached the electrodes do not peel away from the chest.

To summarise:

● V1 Fourth intercostal space at the right sternal border
● V2 Fourth intercostal space at the left sternal border
● V3 Equidistant between V2 and V4
● V4 Fifth intercostal space in the midclavicular line
● V5 Anterior axillary line horizontal with V4
● V6 Midaxillary line horizontal with V4.

ECG cables

Once all of the electrodes have been placed you can then attach the ECG cables. As mentioned previously, the cables connect to the electrodes via clips or studs. Note that the term "cable" and "lead" are interchangeable in ECG-speak and this sometimes causes confusion. The term cable will be used here for clarity. It is perhaps more systematic if you attach the cables in the same order as you placed the electrodes, but in practice it doesn't really matter. What does matter, though, is that the cables are arranged in an orderly fashion across the patient with the acquisition module (the box from which the cables originate) resting somewhere in the middle of the patient. No cables should be dangling loosely from the bed but rather resting neatly on the bed as any movement will be registered as a swinging baseline on the ECG.

ECG cables are generally assigned a colour or a label (and sometimes both) to help the electrocardiographer differentiate between them relatively easily (Table 2.2).

Table 2.2 ECG cable common labels

Cable/electrode position	Colour	Common label(s)
RA	Red	R
LA	Yellow	L
LL	Green	F
RL	Black	N
V1	Red	V1 or C1
V2	Yellow	V2 or C2
V3	Green	V3 or C3
V4	Brown	V4 or C4
V5	Black	V5 or C5
V6	Pink or purple	V6 or C6

Note that the cables are also labelled on the acquisition module and it is therefore possible to trace the intended location of the cable from its origin. Typically the limb cables are located on the outer edges of the module (with the left-sided cables on the right and the right-sided cables on the left). The chest cables then run numerically through the middle. This is really not difficult stuff but it's worthwhile familiarising yourself with the ECG machines and leads in your area before you use them.

Once all of the cables have been attached to the electrodes you should take a few moments to enter the patient details onto the ECG machine. It is suggested that you do this at this point because it allows the electrodes and cables time to settle. Electrodes, by their very nature, require a bit of time after application for a reaction at the skin–electrode interface to take place. You should now be ready to record your ECG. At this point the patient will invariably utter "Looks like I'm wired for sound!" Remember, no matter how many times you hear it, it's still funny.

The ECG machine

Most ECG machines these days provide an automated interpretation of the ECG data. These analysis programs can provide accurate heart rate and conduction interval information. But beware. They are less accurate when it comes to interpretation. Hence they have a tendency to overreport such abnormalities as septal or anterior myocardial infarction and cannot reliably differentiate normal variants and some atrial arrhythmias. Bear in mind then that computer-based ECG interpretation has its uses, but it should not be wholly relied upon to provide a diagnosis.

Standard calibration

ECG machines are universally calibrated to the American Heart Association standard. A common pitfall when looking at an ECG is to get stuck into analysing the rhythm and waveforms without first having a quick look at the calibration settings. Altered calibration settings may superficially resemble ECG abnormalities not relevant to the patient. Any changes in standard calibration that you make during an ECG recording should always be clearly marked on the ECG – however, if you haven't recorded the ECG yourself don't always assume that this has been done for you. Nearly all ECG recorders these days will print calibration settings on the trace.

Sensitivity settings

The calibration mark representing the sensitivity (or gain) of the ECG machine is printed, usually on the left-hand side of the page at the beginning of each line of ECG and should be two large squares (10 mm) in height (Fig. 2.2). This means that for every millivolt measured from the patient a deflection of 10 mm will be recorded on the trace. For the purposes of ECG recording the terms gain and sensitivity are interchangeable.

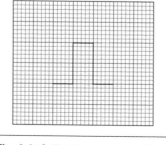

▲ **Fig. 2.2** Calibration mark (sensitivity/gain).

Sensitivity set to 5 mm/mV

Why do it?

In patients with large precordial voltages (as in ventricular hypertrophy) or thin chest walls where the QRS complexes appear to overlap.

What does it look like?

Because setting is half standard calibration all complexes will appear low amplitude.

Not to be confused with...
- Pericardial effusion
- Restrictive cardiomyopathy.

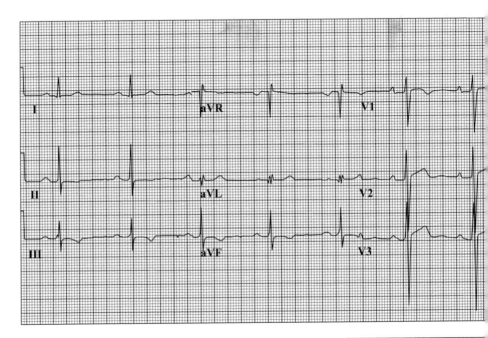

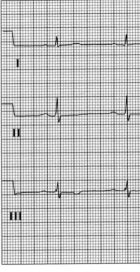

Sensitivity set to 20 mm/mV

Why do it?
To visualise small P waves or other poorly defined complexes.

What does it look like?
Because this setting is at twice the standard calibration setting all complexes will be twice the normal amplitude.

Not to be confused with...
- Left ventricular hypertrophy
- Right atrial enlargement
- Hyperkalaemia.

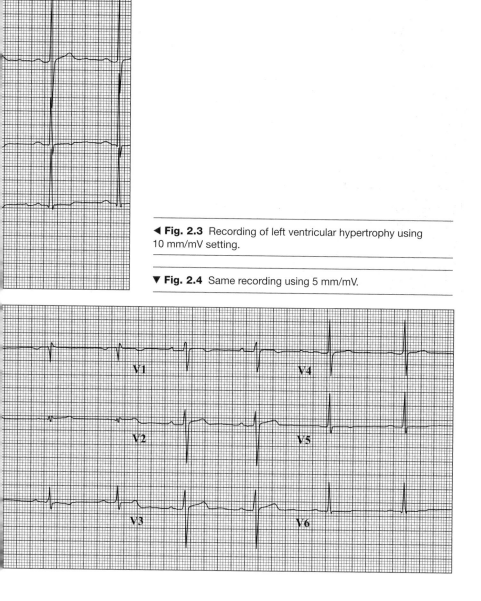

◄ **Fig. 2.3** Recording of left ventricular hypertrophy using 10 mm/mV setting.

▼ **Fig. 2.4** Same recording using 5 mm/mV.

Paper speed settings

Standard paper speed is set to 25 mm/s so that the paper moves through the printer 25 mm every second. Every small square on the ECG paper is therefore equivalent to 0.04 secs (or 40 ms) of time.

Paper speed set to 50 mm/s

Why do it?

In order to determine the presence of P waves during periods of tachycardia. For instance to help differentiate atrial tachyarrhythmias or help decide if a broad complex tachycardia is atrial or ventricular in origin.

What does it look like?

All waveforms and intervals are at twice the standard speed so all appear prolonged.

Not to be confused with...

Any abnormality associated with a prolonged interval. Some examples are:

- Bradycardia
- Left atrial enlargement
- First degree AV block
- Bundle branch block
- Long QT syndrome.

Paper speed set to 5 mm/s or 12.5 mm/s

Why do it?

Rarely used in practice but may be useful when looking for heart-rate changes over time.

What does it look like?

All intervals will be shorter.

Not to be confused with...

- Tachycardia.

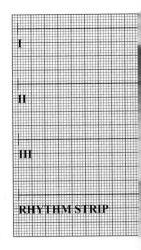

▶ **Fig. 2.5** Diagrammatic format for ECG graph paper.

Filters

All ECG machines have built-in filters so that the range of frequencies classically re-corded is between 0.05–100 Hz. Because other physiological signals (along with extra-neous noise in the environment) also produce frequencies in this range it is sometimes necessary to adjust the filter setting so that the unwanted signals are "filtered out" of our trace. However, filter settings on ECG machines should be adjusted only sparingly when other methods of correcting interference have failed. For unavoidable 50 Hz mains interference – such as when recording an ECG in an intensive care environment – the filter may be switched either "on" or to 40 Hz (depending on what your ECG machine offers as changeable options). It should be noted however, that in doing so all frequen-cies above 40 Hz will be lost from the signal and the resulting ECG signal amplitudes may appear to be less than they really are.

ECG paper

If you look at any sheet of ECG paper you will see it is divided up into around 56 large squares across. You will also see that each large square contains five small squares each equivalent to 1 mm in width. Hence a standard piece of ECG paper is around 280 mm wide.

The ECG, when printed in standard format, is composed of an ECG tracing of all 12 leads divided into four lines of three leads with a continuous rhythm strip (or strips) which is usually printed along the bottom (Fig. 2.5).

Because we know that the paper will move through the printer at a speed of 25 mm in one second we can work out the following:

- Each large square is equivalent to 0.2 seconds
- Each small square is equivalent to 0.04 seconds.

We can therefore also know that:

- Each lead "snapshot" represents 2.5 seconds of time and
- The rhythm strip represents 10 continuous seconds.

Understanding this is important when it comes to calculating heart rate and conduction intervals later on.

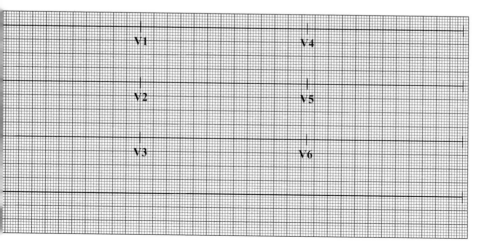

Recognising and reducing artifacts

The term *artifact* refers to any interference or abnormal appearance on an ECG recording that is not due to the measured electrical potentials of the heart. The three most common causes of artifact on an ECG and their remedies are as follows.

Muscle tremor (somatic tremor)

Classically irregular "spiky" oscillations of the baseline.

The ECG in Fig. 2.7 below shows how muscle tremor artifact, if not corrected, may mimic cardiac abnormalities.

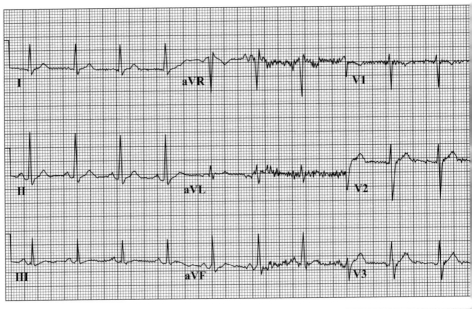

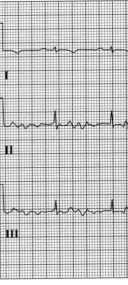

▶ **Fig. 2.7** Muscle tremor and patient movement mimicking atrial flutter.

Table 2.3 Cause and solution for muscle tremor artifact

Cause	Solution
Patient is tense	Ask patient to relax Provide reassurance
Patient is cold	Ensure room is warm Provide blankets if necessary
Patient has Parkinson's disease	Move limb electrodes closer to the torso Ask the patient to tuck their hands under their body

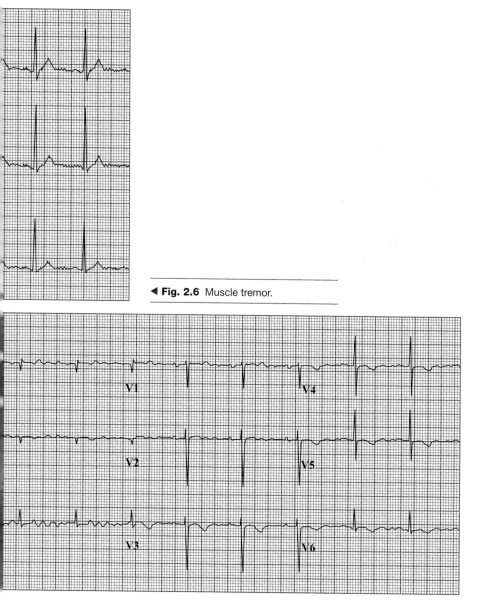

◀ **Fig. 2.6** Muscle tremor.

Table 2.4 Cause and solution for baseline sway artifact

Cause	Solution
Patient is too hot (perspiring)	Ensure room is not too warm. Wipe the skin with an alcohol wipe, dry, then re-apply electrodes
Movement of cable	Ensure cables are not dangling over edge of couch
Respiratory swing (often due to orthopnoea or COPD)	Ask patient to briefly hold breath. If the patient is short of breath give another pillow or adjust bed to a more upright position

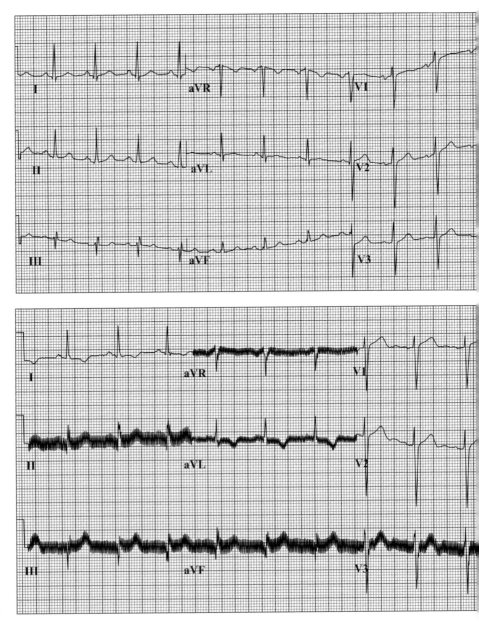

Table 2.5 Cause and solution for AC mains interference artifact

Cause	Solution
Fracture of wire within cable	Check leads and change if necessary
Other electrical equipment	Switch off all non-essential equipment Note: first seek advice if in an intensive care or ward environment

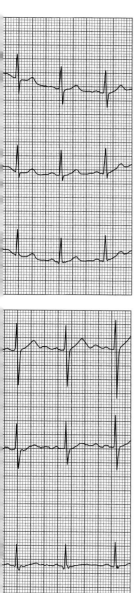

Baseline sway

The tracing wanders across the page and a steady baseline cannot be established.

◀ **Fig. 2.8** Baseline sway.

Mains interference

Regular sinusoidal oscillations of the baseline caused by 50 Hz electrical interference.

◀ **Fig. 2.9** AC mains interference.

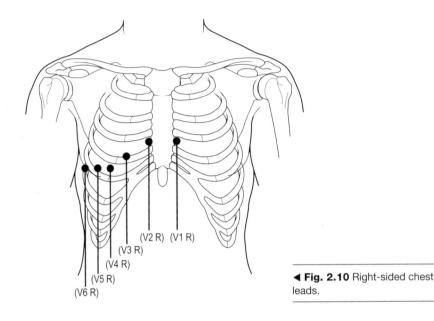

(V2 R) (V1 R)
(V3 R)
(V4 R)
(V5 R)
(V6 R)

◀ **Fig. 2.10** Right-sided chest leads.

Special considerations
It might be necessary, on occasion, to record additional leads on your ECG or to modify your normal practice to suit the patient or circumstances. Some examples are given below.

Recording additional leads

Children
The heart of a child is more centrally placed in the thorax and, in the case of the neonate, there is right ventricular dominance. In children and neonates it is therefore necessary to record at least one right-sided chest lead.

Usually the lead recorded is either V3R or, more commonly, V4R. V4R is found in the midclavicular line in the fifth intercostal space but on the right side of the chest. Whichever cable was used to record the right-sided lead should be labelled accordingly on the ECG. In practice the cable used is the cable usually employed to record lead V1.

This means placing the V1 cable in the V4R position (as shown above). The V2 cable will then be placed in the V1 position on the child's chest. The V3 cable will be placed in the V2 position. Cables V4–V6 should be placed in their normal positions. It is permissible to omit lead V3 from the recording as this will not adversely alter the overall diagnostic value of the ECG. Standard calibration is used although occasionally high amplitude ECG complexes require the sensitivity setting to be reduced to 5 mm/mV. All changes should be clearly marked on the ECG.

Patients with dextrocardia
In dextrocardia the heart lies on the right side of the chest instead of the left. Right-sided chest leads should be recorded in order to accurately record "left ventricular"

Hints and Tips
- Reversal of the arm leads may superficially mimic dextrocardia. In this case lead I will show inverted complexes but chest lead progression will be normal.

complexes. For a comparison of right and left-sided leads recorded in a patient with dextrocardia see page 109.

Patients with acute right ventricular or posterior myocardial infarction

Right ventricular infarction is associated with around 40% of inferior infarctions but is often overlooked because the standard 12 lead ECG does not demonstrate it. Lead V4R should be additionally recorded in patients presenting with acute inferior MI as soon as possible because acute changes in RV MI are often transient. For the sake of speed and accuracy an electrode should be additionally placed in the V4R position during initial electrode placement. A standard 12 lead ECG should first be recorded and then the cable used for the recording of the V4 position may be used to also record V4R for a subsequent ECG. Again, the V4 lead on this second ECG should be clearly marked V4R.

Acute posterior MI is also often missed because the standard 12 lead ECG does not include posterior leads. In patients presenting with suspected posterior MI precordial leads V7 to V9 should additionally be recorded (Fig. 2.11).

All posterior leads are recorded in the same horizontal plane as V4 in the following positions:

- V7 posterior axillary line
- V8 in the mid-scapular line
- V9 recorded at the edge of the spine.

In order to do this you will have to get the patient to turn further onto one side and then swap the cables from the V4, V5 and V6 positions to record V7, V8 and V9. The ECG, of course, should then be labelled accordingly. The fact that this can be a bit tricky is probably the reason why it is not performed routinely in practice.

Modifying standard practice

Patients in wheelchairs

Occasionally you will encounter patients who are wheelchair-bound and, as such, are unable to get up onto a couch or bed. Recording an ECG in these patients is quite straightforward. Skin preparation should be conducted in the usual way and all of the electrodes should be placed in the standard positions. The only complication is the potential for increased somatic tremor on the recording because the patient will have both feet resting either on the ground or footrest and arms leaning on the arm rails. This

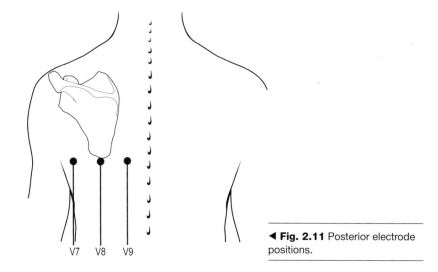

V7 V8 V9

◀ **Fig. 2.11** Posterior electrode positions.

33

can be minimised by placing the leg electrodes on the sides of the knees and the arm electrodes on the upper arms. Asking the patient to hang their arms over the sides of the wheelchair also helps. The ECG should then be recorded as normal with a note stating that the patient was sitting upright for the test.

Patients with amputations and congenital limb abnormalities

Amputation often involves only the partial removal of a limb as in knee or elbow disarticulations. Occasionally, though, it is necessary for whole of the limb to be removed. Also some congenital deformities result in significant shortening of certain limbs. Altering the position of the limb electrodes in these patients may therefore be unavoidable.

Usually, if amputation or deformity is not radical, electrodes may be placed either on the stump or in a position on the affected limbs as far away from the torso as possible. If the right leg has been amputated the electrode may be placed in any other suitable position as this will not affect the cardiac axis. Again, the ECG should be clearly marked to show that the electrode was not in the standard position.

Infectious (or isolated) patients

Anyone who practices electrocardiography is able to contribute to the spread of in-hospital infection due to the portability of the equipment particularly in the presence of poor standards of cleanliness and hygiene. Your own clinical environment will have in place its own local policy with regard to dealing with infectious patients. These should be adhered to at all times. In general an apron and gloves should be worn. Some areas may also stipulate the wearing of a protective mask but any precautions taken should be relevant to the patient and to the threat of cross-infection.

Following contact with an infectious patient all disposables, such as gloves, electrodes etc. should be disposed of, the machine and patient cable should be cleaned using either alcohol or another appropriate disinfectant and your hands should be thoroughly washed *before you leave the room*.

AMBULATORY ECG MONITORING

The ECG can provide useful information when used on the ambulatory patient and is indicated in the following circumstances.

- The assessment and diagnosis of heart rhythm abnormalities in patients presenting with recurrent palpitations, syncope or near-syncope
- The effects of drug therapy
- In patients with neurological symptoms in whom transient atrial fibrillation or flutter is suspected
- Assessment of heart rate variability in patients with hypertrophic cardiomyopathy and heart failure
- In patients with permanent pacemakers to detect pacemaker malfunction and pacemaker-mediated tachycardias.

Monitor types

Ambulatory monitors are predominantly of two types:

- Continuous or
- Intermittent.

The frequency of patient symptoms should dictate the type of monitor selected.

Continuous recorders are suitable for recording periods of between 24 to 48 hours and are useful for the detection of symptoms of a relatively frequent nature. Most continuous recorders include either three or four patient cables, providing two or three channels of ECG.

Intermittent recorders (otherwise known as loop or event recorders) are useful for symptoms that occur infrequently and may be worn for seven days or more. Some may even be activated by the patient at the time of symptoms. However, there are a number of drawbacks:

- They are less useful in syncope with no warning
- They cannot reliably differentiate artifact from cardiac arrhythmias and are therefore prone to the over-counting of "events"
- They can only store a pre-programmed number of events in memory
- They often provide only one channel of ECG
- They provide no information about arrhythmia duration.

Perhaps the biggest advancement in this area has been the relatively recent introduction of the implantable loop recorder. This measures approximately 6 cm by 2 cm and is implanted subcutaneously under local anaesthetic. These monitors may be patient activated via a small hand-held device and are able to present ECG data up to 40 minutes before and two minutes after an event. The obvious advantages of such a system is that they aren't prone to the usual external artifacts like conventional systems and can remain in place for up to 18 months.

The patient diary

The whole point of ambulatory monitoring is to be able to relate the symptoms experienced by a patient to the ECG recording. Hence the use of a patient diary is vitally important.

Ambulatory monitoring is most useful when the patient documents their typical symptoms and this is correlated with an arrhythmia capable of producing such symptoms on the ECG recording. If typical symptoms occur but no abnormality is seen this is enough to demonstrate that the symptoms are unrelated to the heart rhythm and the patient can be reassured. The test is considered equivocal when the patient remains asymptomatic but arrhythmias are documented on the recording. Ambulatory monitoring is least useful when the patient reports no symptoms and the recording is entirely normal. These patients warrant further investigation.

THE ECG AND EXERCISE TESTING

The ECG exercise test is an effective non-invasive procedure providing valuable diagnostic and prognostic information. It is easy to perform, relatively low cost and easily reproducible providing standard protocols are followed. Used appropriately exercise testing is a comparatively low risk procedure with MI or death reported in around 1 in 2500 tests.

Indications for exercise testing

- Assessment of recurrent chest pain in patients with known ischaemic heart disease (IHD) or previous stable angina
- To exclude ischaemic heart disease in patients presenting with atypical chest pain
- Risk stratification in unstable angina and post-myocardial infarction
- Assessment of exercise-induced arrhythmias
- Assessment of the efficacy of interventions such as drug therapy, percutaneous coronary intervention (PCI) or coronary artery bypass grafting (CABG)
- Pre-operative assessment in patients with a history of IHD.

Contraindications to exercise testing

Contraindications fall into two categories: *Absolute* (where the exercise test should not be performed) and *relative* (where the exercise test may be performed with caution. In these circumstances the test should be supervised by a senior doctor).

Absolute contraindications

- Acute myocardial infarction (less than five days ago)
- High risk unstable angina
- Uncontrolled arrhythmias causing symptoms or haemodynamic compromise
- Symptomatic severe aortic stenosis
- Uncontrolled symptomatic heart failure
- Acute pulmonary embolus or pulmonary infarction
- Acute myocarditis or pericarditis
- Acute aortic dissection.

Relative contraindications

- Left main stem coronary stenosis
- Moderate stenotic valvular heart disease
- Electrolyte abnormalities (with ECG changes)
- Uncontrolled hypertension
- Tachyarrhythmias or bradyarrhythmias
- Hypertrophic cardiomyopathy and any other form of outflow obstruction
- Mental or physical impairment leading to inability to exercise adequately
- High degrees of AV block (i.e. second or third degree heart block).

Exercise protocols

A number of protocols are currently available but by far the most widely used are the full and modified Bruce protocols.

A full Bruce protocol comprises seven stages, each stage lasting for three minutes with increasing speed and slope at every stage. The total time for the test, then, is 21 minutes but it is extremely unlikely that a cardiac patient will ever achieve this!

The modified Bruce protocol has two additional stages built in at the beginning with a set speed for the first three stages. As Table 2.7 demonstrates, stage 3 of the modified Bruce protocol is equivalent to stage 1 of the full Bruce. Modified protocols are most often chosen for patients with limited mobility or for the purposes of risk stratification in unstable angina or post-MI.

Note that the use of METS values in these protocols are arbitrarily assigned based on the amount of time, the speed of walking and the slope of the treadmill assuming a standard basal metabolic rate for all patients. In clinical practice you will, of course, encounter patients of different body size, age and sex and so these derived METS values should be interpreted with this in mind.

Table 2.6 The full Bruce protocol

Stage	Time/mins	Speed/mph	Slope/%	METS
1	3	1.7	10	4
2	3	2.5	12	7
3	3	3.4	14	10
4	3	4.2	16	13
5	3	5.0	18	17
6	3	5.5	20	20
7	3	6.0	22	23

Table 2.7 The modified Bruce protocol

Stage	Time/mins	Speed/mph	Slope/%	METS
1	3	1.7	0	1.7
2	3	1.7	5	2.8
3	3	1.7	10	5.0
4	3	2.5	12	7.0
5	3	3.4	14	9.0–10.0
6	3	4.2	16	13.0–14.0
7	3	5.0	18	16.7
8	3	5.5	20	19.0–20.0
9	3	6.0	22	23.0

Test procedure: performing and interpreting an exercise test

Appropriate skin preparation should be performed as for standard 12 lead ECG record-ing. Electrodes should be positioned according to the Mason–Likar modification with limb electrodes sited on the torso. Bear in mind that this will affect the cardiac axis which will undergo a rightward shift.

A pre-test baseline ECG and blood pressure should then be recorded and assessed. Once the test has commenced the ECG should be monitored continuously, the blood pressure recorded every three minutes and the patient observed for adverse signs (i.e. pain, dyspnoea, dizziness, cyanosis etc.) The test should be terminated once the patient has attained their target heart rate (calculated as 220 – patient age) or once another end-point has been reached (see below).

A recovery period should be included during which time the patient should continue to be monitored and until symptoms, ECG changes or blood pressure have returned to baseline values.

A short report should then be written and should include the following points:

- Exercise endpoint (reason for stopping the test)
- Presence of patient symptoms
- Presence of ischaemic ECG changes
- Presence of arrhythmias
- Heart rate and blood pressure response
- Test interpretation (i.e. positive, negative or equivocal).

Exercise endpoints

Endpoints, like contraindications, fall into two categories: absolute and relative.

Absolute endpoints

- Drop in systolic blood pressure of greater than 10 mmHg from baseline despite increasing effort with evidence of ischaemia
- Moderate to severe angina
- Increasing nervous system symptoms (including dizziness or near-syncope)
- Signs of poor perfusion (cyanosis or pallor)
- Technical difficulties in monitoring ECG or systolic blood pressure
- Patient's desire to stop
- Sustained ventricular tachycardia
- ST elevation of greater than 1 mm in leads without diagnostic Q waves*.

*ST elevation in leads with evidence of old infarction (i.e. with pre-existing pathological Q waves) during exercise is thought to be due to underlying regional heart wall motion abnormalities. It is not considered to be evidence of reinfarction.

Relative endpoints

- Drop in systolic blood pressure of greater than 10 mmHg from baseline despite increasing effort without evidence of ischaemia
- ST or QRS changes such as excessive ST depression (greater than 2 mm horizontal or downsloping ST depression) or marked axis shift
- Other arrhythmias including increasing multifocal ventricular ectopy, sustained supraventricular tachycardia, high degrees of heart block or bradyarrhythmias
- Fatigue, shortness of breath, wheezing, leg cramps or claudication
- Development of bundle branch block
- Increasing chest pain
- Hypotensive response.

Heart rate response

Chronotropic incompetence is defined as a failure to reach 85% of the target heart rate despite maximal effort.

Heart rate recovery is considered abnormal if there is less than a 12 bpm decrease in heart rate from peak exercise at two minutes into the recovery period.

Blood pressure response

A rise in systolic blood pressure to greater than 214 mmHg in the normotensive patient is considered to be a hypertensive response. Additionally, BP remaining elevated after three minutes of recovery is also considered a sign of hypertension. A rise in diastolic blood pressure on exercise is associated with coronary artery disease and labile hypertension. Note that severe systemic hypertension may be the cause of arrhythmias (particularly atrial fibrillation) during exercise and exercise-induced ST depression in the absence of ischaemic heart disease.

Hypotensive response is defined as a drop of 20 mmHg or more in systolic blood pressure despite an initial rise or a fall in systolic blood pressure to below the pre-test standing value.

Presence of patient symptoms

Typical anginal chest pain which occurs during exercise and which is associated with ischaemic ECG changes is strongly indicative of underlying ischaemic heart disease. Anginal-type chest pain experienced on exercise but which is not associated with any significant ECG changes does not exclude ischaemic heart disease as the cause but makes it less likely.

Shortness of breath on exertion is a variant form of angina. The test is diagnostic if the patient experiences increasing dyspnoea that is associated with significant ST depression.

Presence of arrhythmias

Increasing ventricular ectopics with exercise, especially if multifocal or occurring as couplets, triplets, salvos and runs of ventricular tachycardia are an indirect marker for ischaemia. Ventricular ectopics present at rest which disappear with exercise is seen to occur in the normal heart.

Interpretation of ST changes

In line with British Cardiac Society guidelines tests are defined as:

- *Positive* – horizontal or downsloping ST segment depression of ≥1 mm or ST elevation in leads without Q waves, measured 80 ms post-J point
- *Negative* – a normal heart rate and blood pressure response with no morphological

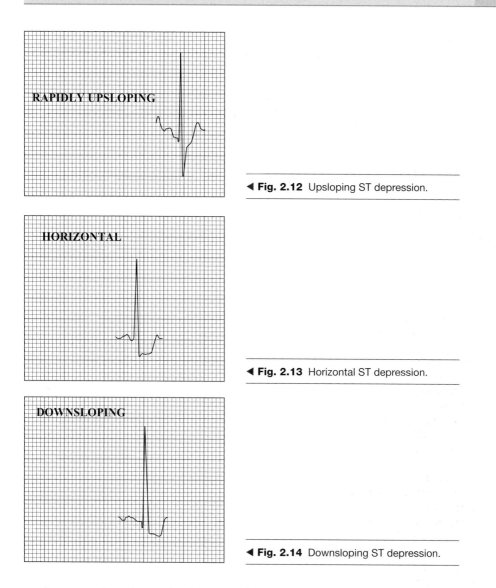

◀ **Fig. 2.12** Upsloping ST depression.

◀ **Fig. 2.13** Horizontal ST depression.

◀ **Fig. 2.14** Downsloping ST depression.

changes and no chest pain, despite attaining at least 85% of the target heart rate
* *Equivocal* – no ST segment changes but 85% of target heart rate not reached.

ST depression is measured 80 milliseconds (or two small squares) post-J point at the level of the PR interval. The J point of a QRS complex is found at the junction of the S wave and ST segment.

Rapidly upsloping ST segment depression is considered a normal finding. Horizontal or downsloping ST depression, however, are considered strongly suggestive of ischaemic heart disease.

Factors affecting test performance and interpretation
The exercise test has a pretty respectable sensitivity (68%) and specificity (77%) but its accuracy is adversely affected by a number of factors.

Test performance may be affected by the actions of certain drugs. Digoxin is thought to produce exercise-induced ST depression in 25–40% of normal healthy subjects. Beta blockers may reduce the diagnostic accuracy of the test by producing an inadequate heart rate response. Antihypertensives affect the haemodynamic response of the patient and nitrates may prevent the patient experiencing their typical anginal symptoms and attenuate the ischaemic response to exercise. There is also an association between flecanide and exercise-induced ventricular tachycardia.

Interpretation of the exercise ECG is affected by any resting ECG abnormality which makes interpretation of the test unreliable or impossible.

Conduction abnormalities such as left bundle branch block (LBBB) render the ECG uninterpretable for ischaemia. Myocardial perfusion scans are a better option for the detection of ischaemia in these patients. Patients with pre-test left bundle branch block may be exercised, in the known absence of ischaemic heart disease, if the test is for the assessment of exercise tolerance. A normal pre-test ECG which develops into rate-dependent left bundle branch block on exercise is an indirect marker of ischaemia.

Right bundle branch block (RBBB) on the resting ECG does not preclude the detection of ischaemia, with ST changes seen in the inferolateral leads having similar accuracy as a normal resting ECG. However, ST depression occurring in leads V1–V4 is common in RBBB and is not associated with ischaemia.

The exercise test is used in patients with Wolf–Parkinson–White syndrome to evaluate the risk of developing rapid ventricular responses during atrial arrhythmias. The abrupt loss of the delta wave at a particular heart rate during exercise implies that it is unlikely that a rapid ventricular response will occur at heart rates above this rate. However, false-positive ST segment depression may occur secondary to accessory pathway conduction.

Patients in atrial fibrillation will demonstrate an abnormal heart rate response during exercise with erratic rises which make the use of the target heart rate as an endpoint unhelpful. Further, patients in AF who are being treated with digoxin may already have marked resting ST depression making further interpretation of the ST segment for ischaemia unreliable.

The presence of left ventricular hypertrophy with typical "strain" pattern on the resting ECG is associated with reduced specificity (sensitivity in these patients is unaffected).

Resting ST depression has been used as a marker for adverse cardiac events in patients without known coronary artery disease especially when a further 2 mm of ST depression or 1 mm of downsloping depression is observed on exercise.

Lists of contraindications and endpoints adapted from the AHA/ACC Guidelines Update for Exercise Testing (2002).

How to read an ECG

HOW TO USE THIS CHAPTER

This chapter provides a practical approach to ECG interpretation and is set out in a way which corresponds to the order in which an ECG should be interpreted in practice. Every time you look at an ECG you should be asking the following three questions.

- What is the heart rate?
- What is the rhythm?
- Are all of the intervals and waveforms within normal limits?

This chapter is divided into three sections to help you to answer these questions.

Section 3.1 Heart rate and rhythms

In this section you will learn how to find the heart rate in both regular and irregular rhythms and how to convert heart rates into time intervals. All of the cardiac rhythms you are likely to encounter are then described. The main body of the text details the aetiology of the rhythm. Each section also includes at least one rhythm strip so you can learn what to expect when you see the rhythm along with several key features. These key features are really all you need to remember, bearing in mind that rhythm identification is quite often a process of simple pattern recognition.

Section 3.2 Intervals and waveforms

Section 2 is to help you assess all of the intervals and waveforms in a straightforward, logical manner. The text is set out as a series of flow charts. Each chart corresponds to a particular ECG waveform or interval, (for example, P waves) describes what might be wrong (i.e. too tall, too wide etc.) and points you in the direction of the associated abnormalities and causes (e.g. right atrial enlargement, left atrial enlargement etc.).

Section 3.3 A–Z of abnormalities

This section deals, in alphabetical order, with all of the corresponding abnormalities so that, having identified that the P waves are too tall, you can immediately look up right atrial enlargement, described in more detail, under "R" (logical, isn't it?). If there is more than one possible cause of the abnormality these will also be listed in alphabetical order.

By placing all of the possible abnormalities in alphabetical order this section can just as easily be used for quick-look reference and provides a multidirectional approach to ECG problems – i.e. starting with an ECG finding and looking up the abnormality which causes it or starting with an abnormality and finding out what changes it can cause on an ECG.

In this way you don't *have* to remember everything, but rather can use the book to *guide* you to the correct diagnosis.

3.1
Heart rate and rhythms

INTRODUCTION

Cardiac rhythms may be broadly described as sinus, atrial, AV junctional or ventricular in origin. There are six key questions you should ask yourself when attempting to identify these rhythms.

1. What is the heart rate?
   Consider both the atrial and ventricular rates and how they relate to one another.
2. Is there evidence of atrial activity?
   This means P waves and flutter or fibrillation waves.
3. Do all of the P waves (if present) occur in the right place?
   P waves preceding the QRS complex are consistent with sinus or atrial rhythms.
   P waves following the QRS complex suggest AV junctional or ventricular rhythms.
4. Are all of the P waves the right shape and right way up?
   P waves differing in configuration from sinus P waves are ectopic in origin.
   Upright P waves in lead II are sinus or atrial in origin. Inverted P waves are always caused by AV junctional or ventricular rhythms.
5. Is the rhythm regular or irregular?
   A fixed irregularity suggests, among other causes, the presence of either sinoatrial or second degree AV block. It is also a feature of certain regularly occurring ventricular arrhythmias such as bigeminy and trigeminy. An irregularity which does not follow any consistent pattern (irregularly irregular) is consistent with atrial fibrillation, flutter or multifocal atrial rhythms.
6. Is the QRS complex broad or narrow?
   If the QRS complex is broad you should consider the possibility of pre-existing bundle branch block, Wolf–Parkinson–White syndrome, aberrant conduction or a rhythm that is ventricular in origin. Narrow complex rhythms are always supraventricular in origin. Note that the term *supraventricular* encompasses both atrial and AV junctional rhythms and so, in literal terms, refers to any rhythm originating from above the ventricles. In practice, however, when describing these rhythms, it is more useful to try and be as specific as possible.

Table 3.1 Cardiac rhythms

Sinus rhythms	Atrial rhythms	Atrioventricular rhythms	Ventricular rhythms
Sinus rhythm	Atrial ectopics	AV junctional rhythms	Ventricular ectopics
Sinus bradycardia	Wandering atrial	AV block	Ventricular tachycardia
Sinus tachycardia	pacemaker	AV re-entrant rhythms	Torsades de pointes
Sinus arrhythmia	Atrial tachycardia		Idioventricular rhythm
Sinus arrest	Multifocal atrial		Ventricular fibrillation
Sinoatrial block	tachycardia		
	Atrial fibrillation		
	Atrial flutter		

All of the rhythms listed in Table 3.1 above are described in the following pages. Additionally, cardiac arrest, peri-arrest and pacemaker rhythms are also described.

HOW TO FIND THE HEART RATE

You will remember from Chapter 2 that ECG graph paper is divided into big squares and small squares. You will also know that the speed at which the paper moves through the printer is at a rate of 25 mm each second. This means that:

- Each large square is equivalent to 0.2 seconds
- Each small square is equivalent to 0.04 seconds.

From these basic principles it is possible to calculate the heart rate. You should note that the examples which follow illustrate finding the ventricular (or QRS) rate. The same principles may be applied, however, when determining the atrial (or P wave) rate.

Finding the heart rate in a regular rhythm

A number of methods exist for heart rate calculations in regular rhythms but by far the two most commonly used are as follows.

Method 1

Count the number of large squares between two consecutive QRS complexes and divide into 300.

$$\text{Method 1} \quad \frac{300}{\text{Number of large squares}}$$

This method has the advantage of being quick and easy. However, it amounts only to an estimate unless you are able to find two consecutive QRS complexes falling exactly on the boundaries between the large squares. The basis for this method is that a one-minute strip of ECG covers 300 large squares. Remember that heart rate is expressed in beats per minute.

Method 2

Although the "quick look" method above will provide you with an approximate heart rate it may sometimes be necessary to provide a heart rate that is more accurate. The second method is a bit more long-winded but more accurate than the first and involves counting the number of small squares between two consecutive QRS complexes and then dividing into 1500.

$$\text{Method 2} \quad \frac{1500}{\text{Number of small squares}}$$

The basis for this method is that a one-minute strip of ECG will cover 1500 small squares. You should be able to see that the longer way is more accurate because the rates we produce are more discrete, that is, they are not convenient round numbers.

Finding the heart rate in an irregular rhythm

Because of the variability in R–R intervals in irregular rhythms you need to take account of a larger number of complexes over which to calculate your heart rate so that what you're getting is an average. You can do this simply by counting out 30 large squares (from any starting point on the rhythm strip) and then counting the number of QRS complexes within that 30 squares and multiplying by 10.

Method 3

Number of QRS complexes in 30 large squares x 10.

Table 3.2 Heart rate calculation method 1

Number of large squares (between two R waves)	Heart rate/ bpm
1	300
1.5	200
2	150
3	100
4	75
5	60
6	50
7	45
8	40
9	35
10	30

Table 3.3 Heart rate calculation method 2

Number of small squares (between two R waves)	Heart rate/ bpm
5	300
6	250
7	214
8	188
9	167
10	150
11	136
12	125
13	115
14	107
15	100
16	94
17	88
18	83
19	79
20	75
21	71
22	68
23	65
24	62
25	60

▼ **Fig. 3.1** Using method 1 we can see that the number of large squares is roughly equivalent to four and a bit (see arrows). Four large squares would give us a heart rate of 75 bpm, so lets say the heart rate is 70 bpm (allowing for the bit). Using method 2 we can see that the number of small squares equals 22. Divide this into 1500 and you should get a heart rate of 68 bpm.

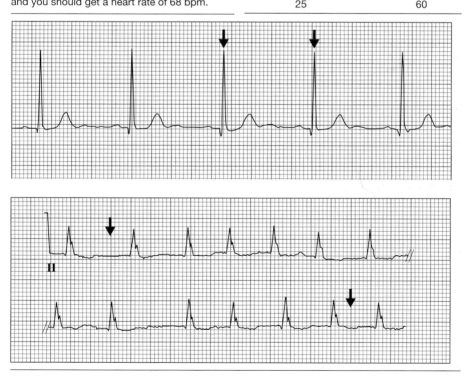

▲ **Fig. 3.2** The number of QRS complexes occurring within the 30 large squares (as marked with arrows on the ECG above) is equal to 13. This gives us an average heart rate of 130 bpm. (Note that the rhythm shown is continuous.)

How to determine if a rhythm is regular

A rhythm is said to be regular if the difference between the longest and shortest R–R intervals is less than 0.16 seconds. This may not always be simple to determine in practice so another, less mathematical, way is to mark the position of two or more R waves on a piece of paper and move the positions along each interval. The marked positions should match up with the R waves all the way along the strip (give or take very minor variations).

Is the heart rate normal?

The heart rate can now be classified as:

- Normal = 60–100 bpm
- Bradycardia = less than 60 bpm
- Tachycardia = greater than 100 bpm.

The normal values above are described for the average adult at rest but in practice this will vary between patients.

The 60 000 rule

It is often useful to convert heart rates into time intervals. For instance suppose you had just recorded an ECG from a patient who was having long pauses in his normal rhythm due to disease of his conduction system. How could you tell just how long the pause lasted?

Firstly you would find the heart rate by either of the methods described above. Say that the number of large squares between the two consecutive R waves incorporating the pause was 15. The heart rate would then be equal to 20 bpm between these two points.

You can now convert the heart rate into a time interval by using the 60 000 rule.

$$\frac{60\ 000}{HR} = \text{time interval in milliseconds}$$

So, 60 000/20 bpm = 3000 ms or 3 seconds (by dividing the answer by 1000).

SINUS RHYTHMS

Normal sinus rhythm

For rhythms originating at the sinus node we should ask ourselves what do we already know about sinus node activity? Well, we know that the sinus node depolarises spontaneously between 60–100 times each minute. We also know this depolarisation travels from top-to-bottom across the atria with a vector towards lead II. Therefore we should expect to see an upright P wave in this lead. In normal sinus rhythm we expect the AV node to conduct the impulse normally, hence we should expect one P wave for every QRS complex.

In thinking this way we have pretty much described the rhythm strip below.

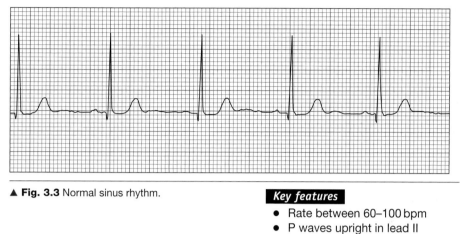

▲ **Fig. 3.3** Normal sinus rhythm.

Key features

- Rate between 60–100 bpm
- P waves upright in lead II
- One P wave for every QRS

Sinus bradycardia

A bradycardia is simply a "slow heart rate". Hence sinus bradycardia is plainly a slow heart rate originating at the sinus node and shares all the key features of normal sinus rhythm except the rate is less than 60 bpm.

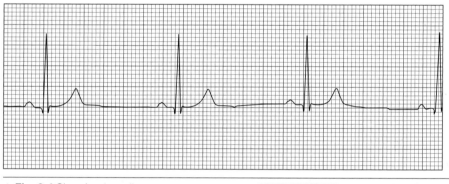

▲ **Fig. 3.4** Sinus bradycardia.

Key features

- Rate less than 60 bpm
- P waves upright in lead II
- One P wave for every QRS

CAUSES

- Athletic hearts
- Drug effects (e.g. beta blockers)
- Electrolyte imbalances
- Hypothermia
- Hypothyroidism
- Sick sinus syndrome
- Sleep.

Sinus tachycardia

A tachycardia simply means "fast heart rate". Hence sinus tachycardia shares all the key features of normal sinus rhythm except with a heart rate in excess of 100 bpm.

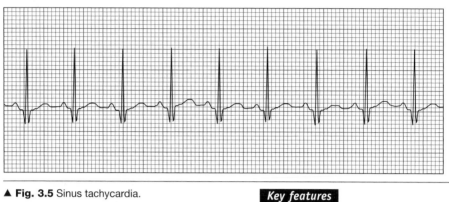

▲ **Fig. 3.5** Sinus tachycardia.

Key features

- Rate more than 100 bpm
- P waves upright in lead II
- One P wave for every QRS

CAUSES

- Anaemia
- Caffeine and other stimulants
- Drug effects (e.g. salbutamol and atropine)
- Exercise and stress
- Fluid loss
- Heart failure
- Normal variant in paediatrics
- Pulmonary embolism
- Thyrotoxicosis.

Inappropriate sinus tachycardia is defined as a persistent increase in resting heart rate unrelated to, or out of proportion with, the level of physical, emotional, pathological or pharmacologic stress. It is thought to be due to enhanced automaticity or abnormal autonomic regulation of the sinus node. Patients are generally females in their mid–late thirties presenting with palpitations, shortness of breath, dizziness, lightheadedness and presyncope.

Another type of inappropriate sinus tachycardia is postural orthostatic tachycardia syndrome (POTS) thought to be caused by autonomic dysfunction which causes the patient to suffer symptoms while standing which are relieved by sitting or lying down. Such symptoms include exercise intolerance, palpitations, weakness and lightheadedness.

Sinus arrhythmia

Sinus arrhythmia is a normal variation in heart rate with an apparent tachycardia during inspiration and a bradycardia during expiration. It is caused by stimulation of the vagus nerve during respiration which supplies the sinus node. Indeed the absence of sinus arrhythmia can be used to diagnose autonomic dysfunction which can be a neuropathic consequence of diseases such as diabetes.

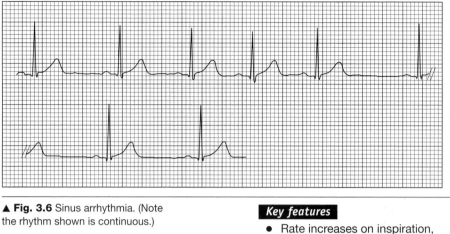

▲ **Fig. 3.6** Sinus arrhythmia. (Note the rhythm shown is continuous.)

Key features

- Rate increases on inspiration, decreases on expiration
- P waves upright in lead II
- One P wave for every QRS

CAUSES

- Increased vagal tone common in the young. Note that when sinus arrhythmia is observed in the elderly it is called idiopathic sinus arrhythmia
- May be a feature of sick sinus syndrome.

Sick sinus syndrome (SSS)

Sick sinus syndrome is caused by impaired sinus node activity leading to abnormalities in both impulse formation and conduction. It largely manifests itself as marked sinus bradycardia but it is also responsible for the appearance of "sinus pauses" (caused by sinus arrest or sinoatrial block) and a phenomenon called bradycardia–tachycardia (brady–tachy) syndrome. So-called escape rhythms are also a feature.

Patients with sick sinus syndrome are commonly elderly and present with a range of symptoms which include syncope, dizzy spells and palpitations. The condition has many potential causes, the main one being idiopathic fibrosis of the sinus node.

ECG findings

Normal sinus rhythm is more often the predominant rhythm in this group of patients with intermittent periods of the following:

Common ECG features

- Marked sinus bradycardia
- Sinoatrial block
- Sinus arrest
- Brady–tachy syndrome
- Escape beats/rhythms.

Sinus bradycardia

Often marked, sinus bradycardia may occur at rates in the region of 30 bpm.

Sinoatrial block

Sinoatrial block is the intermittent failure of the sinus node to activate the atria resulting in a pause on the ECG which is equivalent to – or a multiple of – the cycle length during sinus rhythm. To explain this further look at the example below.

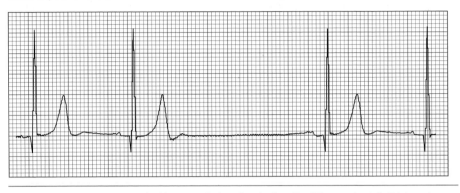

▲ **Fig. 3.7** The pause shown in this example is *twice* the length of the previous P–P interval.

Sinus arrest

Sinus arrest is the failure of the sinus node to activate the atria resulting in a pause on the ECG which bears no relationship to the predominant cycle length. Note that in the case of both sinoatrial block and sinus arrest a P wave fails to appear preceding the pause.

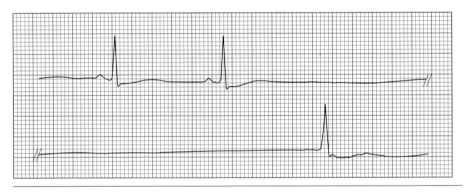

▲ **Fig. 3.8** This ECG shows sinus arrest resulting in a pause of 4.8 seconds. The pause is terminated by a low junctional escape beat. The ECG was taken from a 75-year-old woman admitted via the A&E department after an episode of syncope. She apparently recovered consciousness rapidly, in time to call her husband for help. On questioning she admitted feeling short episodes of palpitations at rest, lasting about two minutes. At times, these palpitations were accompanied by light-headedness. She later went on to receive a permanent pacemaker. (Note that the rhythm shown is continuous.)

Brady–tachy syndrome

This syndrome is so-called because the tachycardias often alternate with the brady-cardia produced by sinus node dysfunction. The most common tachycardias are atrial fibrillation and, less frequently, atrial flutter. Atrial tachycardia may also occur. AV re-entrant tachycardia, though, is not a feature of this syndrome. All of these atrial arrhyth-mias are described in detail in the sections below.

Escape beats and rhythms

Escape rhythms or single escape beats are often seen following a prolonged pause and are a part of the heart's "safety net" of subsidiary pacemakers (see detail on automaticity in Chapter 1). These beats or rhythms will typically be junctional (again, see below) unless the disease also involves the AV junction in which case the escape will be ventricular in origin.

Causes of sick sinus syndrome

- Cardiac surgery
- Cardiomyopathy
- Drug effects (e.g.digoxin or quinidine toxicity)
- Ischaemic heart disease
- Myocarditis
- Sinus node fibrosis.

ATRIAL RHYTHMS

Atrial ectopics

When the atria are depolarised at any point other than at the sinus node an ectopic beat is produced demonstrating a P wave which looks different to the sinus P wave. Any P wave (or depolarisation of the atria) may, in turn, activate the ventricles. The ectopic beat typically occurs earlier than expected in the cycle and is followed by a short compensatory pause.

CAUSES

- Atrial enlargement
- Digitalis toxicity
- Hyperthyroidism

- Ischaemic heart disease
- Mitral valve disease
- Rheumatic heart disease.

Atrial ectopics are often of no clinical significance and occur in structurally normal hearts in small numbers. However, frequent atrial ectopics, especially if associated with tachycardias, may be a sign of underlying heart disease.

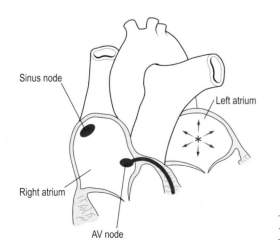

Sinus node

Left atrium

Right atrium

AV node

◀ **Fig. 3.9** Atrial ectopic focus.

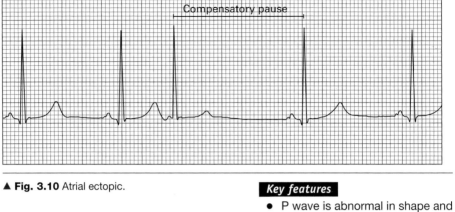

▲ **Fig. 3.10** Atrial ectopic.

Key features

- P wave is abnormal in shape and occurs early
- Normal (narrow) QRS conduction
- Compensatory pause

Occasionally an atrial ectopic will occur while the bundle branches are (still recovering from the previous impulse) refractory and hence conduction through the ventricles does not result. In this case a P wave may appear on the T wave of the preceding beat and a slightly longer R–R interval ensues.

Be cautious as this may be confused by the overzealous with second degree heart block but, unlike heart block, is not an indication for cardiac pacing.

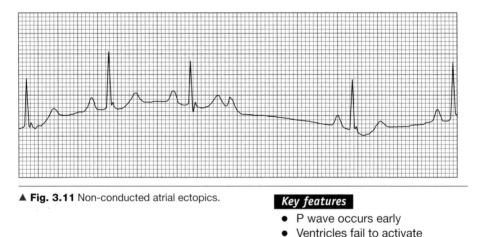

▲ **Fig. 3.11** Non-conducted atrial ectopics.

Key features

- P wave occurs early
- Ventricles fail to activate
- Slightly longer than normal R–R interval

Wandering atrial pacemaker

A wandering atrial pacemaker is really just a lot of atrial ectopics firing off from different parts of the atrial myocardium. The result as far as the ECG is concerned is P waves of variable morphology. Because there is no particular order to the depolarisation the P waves may occur early or late in the cycle giving rise to an irregular-looking QRS rhythm.

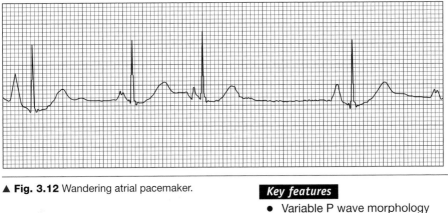

▲ **Fig. 3.12** Wandering atrial pacemaker.

Key features

- Variable P wave morphology
- Variable PR intervals
- Variable R–R intervals
- Heart rate less than 100 bpm

Atrial tachycardia (AT)

Atrial tachycardia is formed by a rapid succession of atrial ectopics and consequently shares similar features to single atrial ectopic beats. This arrhythmia is nearly always a paroxysmal (intermittent) ECG finding and is often referred to as paroxysmal atrial tachycardia (PAT).

CAUSES

- As for atrial ectopics.

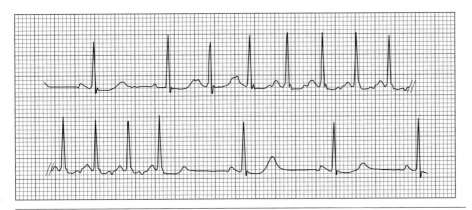

▲ **Fig. 3.13** Atrial tachycardia.

Key features

- First beat occurs early
- Abnormally shaped P waves (which may be upright in lead II)
- Rate greater than 100 bpm (but usually greater than 120 bpm)
- Compensatory pause

Multifocal atrial tachycardia (MAT)

A multifocal atrial tachycardia is, as the name implies, produced by varying ectopic foci within the atria firing off randomly so that the ECG looks like a rapid run of atrial ectopics. Put simply this is wandering atrial pacemaker at a rate greater than 100 bpm. The QRS rate is irregular and fast (and looks a bit like AF but with P waves).

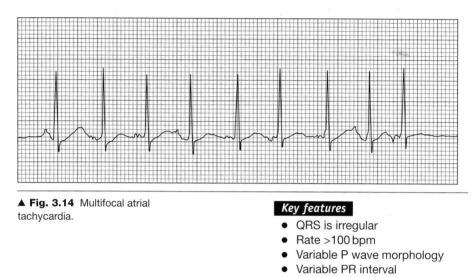

▲ **Fig. 3.14** Multifocal atrial tachycardia.

Key features

- QRS is irregular
- Rate >100 bpm
- Variable P wave morphology
- Variable PR interval

Atrial fibrillation (AF)

The basis for atrial fibrillation is multiple ectopic foci within the atria firing off at rates of up to 600 times a minute. This results in no discernible P wave but rather small ripple-like oscillations known as fibrillation waves. Conduction to the ventricles is said to be "irregularly irregular" due to the refractoriness of the AV node.

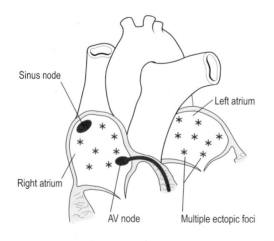

Sinus node

Left atrium

Right atrium

AV node   Multiple ectopic foci

◀ **Fig. 3.15** Multiple atrial ectopic foci in atrial fibrillation.

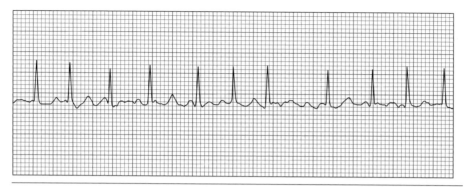

▲ **Fig. 3.16** This ECG was taken from a middle-aged man who had been attending six-monthly appointments at the specialist cardiology clinic for the last three years. He had mitral valve prolapse with significant mitral regurgitation, diagnosed incidentally during a medical check up. During this visit, he complained of a three-week history of fatiguability and shortness of breath on walking uphill.

Key features
- Ripple-like oscillations of the baseline (no discernible P waves)
- QRS rate irregularly irregular

CAUSES ARE DIVIDED AS FOLLOWS

Acute causes and precipitating conditions
- Acute myocardial infarction or angina
- Alcohol intake
- Electrocution
- Hyperthyroidism
- Idiopathic
- Myocarditis
- Post-cardiothoracic surgery
- Pericarditis
- Pneumonia and infective exacerbations of COPD
- Pulmonary embolism
- Rheumatic fever.

Cardiovascular disease associated with a high incidence of AF
- Cardiac tumours such as atrial myxoma
- Cardiomyopathy
- Congenital heart disease especially ASD
- Congestive heart failure
- Constrictive pericarditis
- Cor pulmonale
- Hypertension
- Ischaemic heart disease
- Intrathoracic pathology (e.g. lung cancer, mediastinal tumours etc.)
- Mitral valve stenosis and regurgitation (rheumatic and non-rheumatic causes)
- Myocardial infiltrative diseases such as amyloidosis and haemochromatosis
- Pre-excitation syndromes
- Sick sinus syndrome.

AF nomenclature

Recurrent; more than one episode of AF has occurred.

Valvular; AF occurring in a patient with evidence or history of rheumatic mitral valve disease or prosthetic heart valves.

Paroxysmal; AF that typically lasts seven days or less with spontaneous conversion to sinus rhythm. This does not apply to episodes lasting 30 seconds or less or to episodes precipitated by a reversible medical condition such as myocardial infarction, cardiac surgery, pericarditis, myocarditis, hyperthyroidism, pulmonary embolism, and acute pulmonary disease.

Persistent; AF that typically lasts longer than seven days or requires pharmacologic or direct current DC cardioversion.

Permanent; AF that is refractory to cardioversion and that has persisted for longer than one year.

Lone (or idiopathic); AF occurring in a patient younger than 60 years who has no clinical or echocardiographic evidence of cardiopulmonary disease. This type of AF can be broken down into two further subdivisions: adrenergic (a common sympathetically-mediated form) and vagotonic (a less common vagally-mediated form). These two types may be distinguished by a number of features.

Adrenergic

- Tends to occur in older patients of either sex
- Usually there is evidence of underlying heart disease
- Usually diurnal occurrence
- Triggered by stress, exercise
- Vagal manoeuvres can stop or slow an attack
- Ventricular response is typically fast during periods of AF
- All class I, II, III and IV drugs can be useful.

Vagotonic

- Relatively young, predominantly male patients
- Often no underlying heart disease
- Classically nocturnal occurrence
- Triggered by heavy meals, alcohol, GORD, post-exercise (stress usually not a trigger)
- Occurs in patients with slow heart rates (i.e. athletes)
- Notable features: multiple ectopics preceding attack; increasing HR can prevent attacks; often appears as a combination of fibrillation and flutter
- Vagal manoeuvres can cause an attack
- Ventricular response during AF is slow
- Effective drugs: disopyramide, flecainide
- Contraindicated drugs: digoxin, beta blockers
- Can be identified using HR variability analysis on ambulatory monitoring.

Adapted from the AHA/ACC/ESC Guidelines for the Management of Patients with Atrial Fibrillation: Executive Summary (2001).

Atrial fibrillation is very common among the elderly. AF is capable of producing a slow and rapid ventricular response. Often changes in posture and the onset of exercise or any form of exertion can cause large jumps in heart rate. Heart rate control is therefore the biggest challenge in these patients.

Atrial flutter

Atrial flutter results from one of two mechanisms.

1. An atrial ectopic focus similar to atrial tachycardia but with a much faster atrial (P wave) rate.
2. A self-perpetuating circular path of atrial depolarisation which typically forms a continuous circuit between the inferior and superior vena cavae within the right atrium.

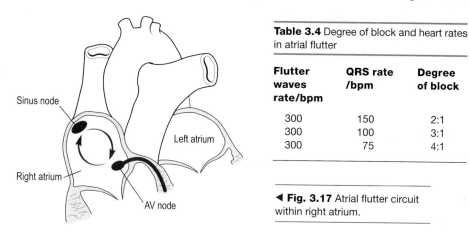

Sinus node

Left atrium

Right atrium

AV node

Table 3.4 Degree of block and heart rates in atrial flutter

Flutter waves rate/bpm	QRS rate /bpm	Degree of block
300	150	2:1
300	100	3:1
300	75	4:1

◄ **Fig. 3.17** Atrial flutter circuit within right atrium.

Circular depolarisation is by far the most common of the mechanisms. Think of it like a Mexican wave. It only takes one madcap football fan to get it started and before you know it the wave has spread from its point of origin (i.e. the madcap fan) all around the stadium and back again. If this wave was to circulate at 250–300 times a minute, you wouldn't be a million miles from atrial flutter (as well as certain exhaustion!).

This rapid rate of atrial stimulation results in "sawtooth" oscillations of the baseline. Because the AV node cannot conduct these impulses through to the ventricles at such a rate an AV block develops, typically (with flutter waves at a rate of 300 bpm) 2:1, 3:1 or 4:1. However, it is not unusual for the degree of block to vary in any one patient presenting with atrial flutter.

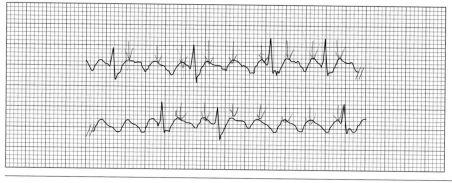

▲ **Fig. 3.18** Atrial flutter: variable block. (Note that the rhythm shown is continuous.)

Key features

- Sawtooth appearance of baseline
- Atrial rate 250–350 bpm (but typically 300 bpm)
- Presence of AV block

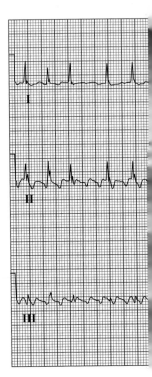

▶ **Fig. 3.19** This ECG shows a sawtooth baseline with ventricular rate of exactly 150 bpm (apart from in the initial portion) typical of atrial flutter with 2:1 block.

If you see a regular atrial tachycardia at a fixed rate of 150 bpm you should think atrial flutter with 2:1 block.

CAUSES

As for atrial fibrillation.

ATRIOVENTRICULAR RHYTHMS

AV junctional rhythms

So-called because they arise from around the AV junction and may involve the AV node and the bundle of His. Because the impulse is formed from around the AV junction the

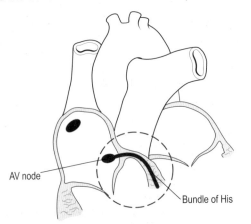

AV node

Bundle of His

◀ **Fig. 3.20** Site of junctional arrhythmias.

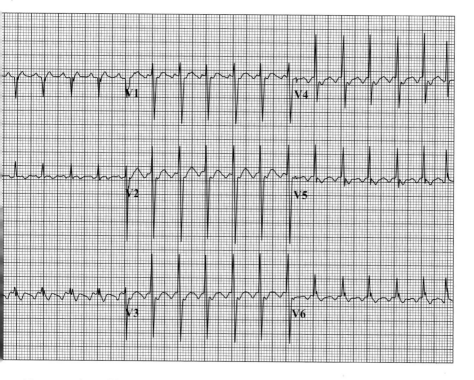

atria are activated in a retrograde (or reverse) direction and so the P wave will be inscribed upside-down on the ECG. Depending on the relative speeds of the retrograde
and anterograde (forward) conduction from the AV junction, the P waves may appear
before, during or after the QRS complexes.

Junctional rhythms are described as being either passive or active. Passively
arising junctional rhythms are essentially escape beats or rhythms brought about by
inadequate sinus node activity. The normal rate of automaticity from around the AV
junction is 45–60 bpm.

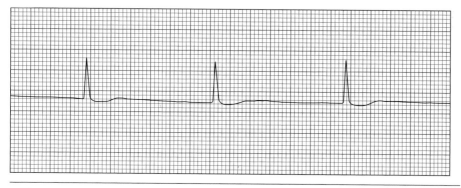

▲ **Fig. 3.21** This ECG shows
a QRS rate of 48 bpm with no
visible P waves (P waves are
occurring *during* the QRS),
consistent with a mid-junctional
escape rhythm.

Key features

• P waves appear before, during or
  after QRS
• P waves appear inverted
• Regular QRS rate between 45–60 bpm

CAUSES

- Sinoatrial block
- Sinus arrest
- Sinus bradycardia
- Second or third degree AV block.

Junctional rhythms that are actively formed tend to produce junctional ectopic beats and tachycardias. Junctional tachycardias are defined as being either paroxysmal (intermittent) or non-paroxysmal (permanent). Paroxysmal junctional tachycardia may occur in normal healthy individuals at rates between 160–250 bpm but is relatively uncommon. Non-paroxysmal tachycardia on the other hand is more commonly seen in organic heart disease and particularly in digitalis toxicity at rates between 60–130 bpm. This is often referred to as an accelerated junctional rhythm.

Atrioventricular (heart) block

Conduction from the atria to the ventricles via the AV node may be either delayed (as in first degree AV block) or blocked. The block may be either transient and intermittent (as in second degree AV block) or permanent (as in third degree or complete AV block). All of the heart blocks described below may be a complication of acute myocardial infarction (especially if the right coronary artery is involved).

CAUSES OF AV BLOCK

- Acute myocardial infarction
- Congenital heart disease
- Cardiomyopathy
- Drugs effects (e.g. digoxin, calcium channel blockers, beta blockers, amiodarone)
- Fibrosis and sclerosis of the conduction system
- Hyperkalaemia
- Increased vagal tone
- Infiltrating malignancies
- Ischaemic heart disease
- Myocarditis
- Valvular disease.

First degree AV block

This is typified by a prolongation of the PR interval to greater than 0.20 seconds (five small squares) as the impulse is conducted slower than normal through the AV node. Transmission to the ventricles occurs with a fixed (1:1) relationship between the P wave and the QRS complex (Fig. 3.22).

First degree AV block does not cause symptoms and does not require treatment *on its own*. Treatment, if indicated, should be focused to the causes (see above).

First degree block is not, in itself, a contraindication to beta-blockers or other negatively inotropic drugs, but higher degrees of block developing as a result of treatment should alert you to the possibility of more serious conductive tissue disease. The development of first degree (or higher) AV block in infective endocarditis may be a sign of an aortic root abscess.

Second degree AV block

There are **three** types of second degree AV block namely:

- Mobitz type I
- Mobitz type II
- 2:1 AV block.

Mobitz type I (Wenckebach phenomenon)

There is a cyclic prolongation of the PR interval starting with a normal PR interval which progressively lengthens until one P wave is not followed by a QRS complex and a pause ensues. The next beat demonstrates a normal PR interval and the cycle begins again.

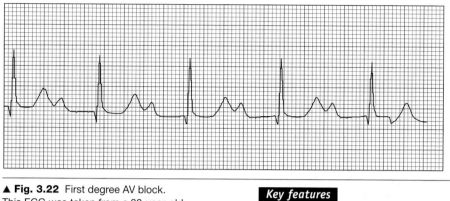

▲ **Fig. 3.22** First degree AV block.
This ECG was taken from a 30-year-old
competitive swimmer and is consistent
with high vagal tone in an athlete.

Key features

- PR interval >0.20 secs (and constant)
- One P wave for every QRS

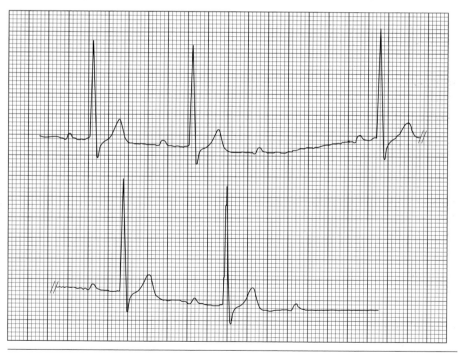

▲ **Fig. 3.23** Mobitz type I
(Wenckebach). (Note rhythm
shown is continuous.)

Key features

- Cyclic prolongation of PR interval leading to a non-conducted P wave

This type of block often occurs during sleep or during periods of high vagal activity. Generally it does not require pacing unless haemodynamic compromise is evidenced

Mobitz type II

This, less common, form of second degree block is characterised by occasional non-conducted P waves.

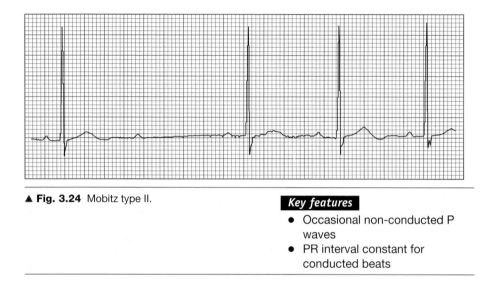

▲ **Fig. 3.24** Mobitz type II.

<table>
<tr><td colspan="2">Key features</td></tr>
<tr><td>●</td><td>Occasional non-conducted P waves</td></tr>
<tr><td>●</td><td>PR interval constant for conducted beats</td></tr>
</table>

2:1 AV block

This third form of second degree heart block is characterised by a fixed ratio of conducted to non-conducted P waves, where two P waves are seen for every one QRS complex.

Note both the Mobitz type II and 2:1 AV block forms of second degree heart block are more frequently associated with symptoms and have a tendency to deteriorate into complete heart block or asystole. Seek advice as pacing may be indicated.

AV dissociation

In AV dissociation the atria and ventricles function independently from one another so that the P waves, fibrillation or flutter waves bear no relationship to the QRS complexes. This can occur in the following circumstances:

● When there is slowing or impairment of the sinus node
● When impulse formation in the AV junction or ventricles is accelerated
● During ventricular mode (VVI) pacing (see pacemaker rhythms).

AV dissociation may be either complete or incomplete. In the case of complete AV dissociation the atria and ventricles operate independently continuously. Incomplete AV dissociation is said to be present whenever there is a relationship (however infrequently) between the atria and ventricles as demonstrated by so-called captured beats. Captured beats may be either ventricular or atrial. Ventricular captured beats are sinus or atrial ectopic impulses which are conducted normally to the ventricles. Atrial captured beats (although less common) are ventricular impulses which may be conducted retrogradely to the atria. AV dissociation in the presence of intermittent

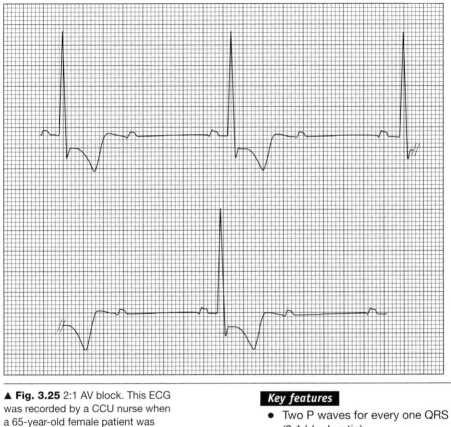

▲ **Fig. 3.25** 2:1 AV block. This ECG was recorded by a CCU nurse when a 65-year-old female patient was noted to have a slow heart rate. The patient had been admitted a few hours previously with an inferior MI. She had been given streptokinase on admission. Her BP was 100/50, and she felt well. (Note rhythm shown is continuous.)

Key features

- Two P waves for every one QRS (2:1 block ratio)
- PR interval constant for conducted beats
- Constant P–P interval

captured beats is termed advanced (or high-degree) AV dissociation and should be distinguished from complete AV block below.

Complete (third degree) heart block (CHB)

In this form of heart block there is no conduction from the atria to the ventricles and the two therefore work entirely independently of each other.

The QRS complex in complete heart block may be either broad or narrow depending on whereabouts the escape rhythm is being generated. Impulses generated high up the conduction system (around the area of the bundle of His or AV junction) will produce a narrow QRS with a faster escape heart rate and are generally better tolerated by patients. Those generated further down (from the ventricular myocardium and Purkinje system) will more likely produce a broader complex with slower resultant heart rates. Complete heart block, particularly if symptomatic, requires pacing and cardiology advice should always be sought.

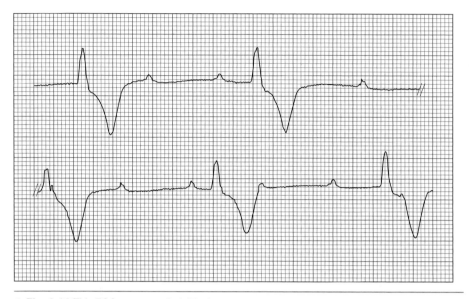

▲ **Fig. 3.26** This ECG was recorded 15 minutes before cardiac arrest. The patient had recently been admitted to the coronary care unit following an anterior MI. He was feeling extremely unwell and short of breath, with a systolic blood pressure of 80 mmHg. The ECG shows sinus rhythm (with a sinus rate of 98 bpm) and complete heart block with a ventricular escape rhythm of 35 bpm. (Note rhythm shown is continuous.)

Key features
- No relationship between atrial and ventricular activity
- PR interval appears variable (because in CHB it doesn't exist!)

Complete heart block with atrial fibrillation

The ECG below shows atrial fibrillation in the presence of complete heart block. At first glance you may be forgiven for thinking this is slow AF but note that the ventricular response is *regular*. Again, the QRS may be either broad or narrow.

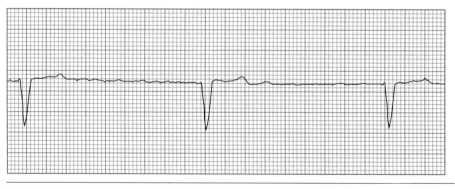

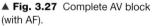

▲ **Fig. 3.27** Complete AV block (with AF).

Key features
- Irregular oscillation of the baseline (fibrillation waves)
- Slow, regular ventricular rate

AV re-entry rhythms

Both AV re-entry and AV nodal re-entry tachycardias require an additional conduction pathway. This pathway is located either within the AV node itself (as in AV nodal re-entry) or completely separate from the AV node (as in AV re-entry).

The mechanisms are similar to the Mexican wave of atrial flutter, in that they form a self-perpetuating circle of depolarisation either round and around the AV node or through the AV node and back to the atria via the additional pathway.

The key to distinguishing AV re-entry from AV nodal re-entry on an ECG lies in the position of the retrograde P wave.

In AV re-entry, the separate accessory pathway provides a larger circuit within which the impulse must travel before the atria are reactivated, therefore the retrograde P wave will often appear midway between two QRS complexes, and often on top of a T wave.

In AV nodal re-entry tachycardia the re-entry circuit is within the AV node itself and the circuit is therefore very small. Hence the retrograde P waves will appear very shortly

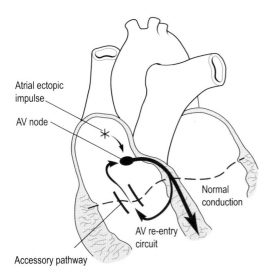

Atrial ectopic impulse

AV node

Normal conduction

AV re-entry circuit

Accessory pathway

◀ **Fig. 3.28** AV re-entry circuit. An impulse travels in an anterograde direction through the AV node to the ventricles as normal but then re-enters the atria via a separate accessory pathway in a retrograde direction.

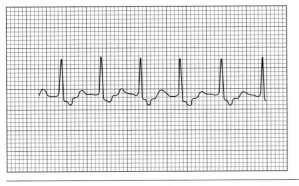

▲ **Fig. 3.29** AV re-entry tachycardia.

Key features

- Retrograde P waves following QRS complexes
- Rate 130–250 bpm

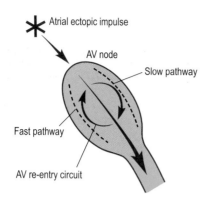

Atrial ectopic impulse

AV node

Slow pathway

Fast pathway

AV re-entry circuit

◀ **Fig. 3.30** AV nodal re-entry circuit. An atrial ectopic impulse is conducted to the AV node at a critical time when the fast-conducting pathway within the AV node is still refractory. The impulse is conducted down the slow pathway and then retrogradely through the fast pathway once it has recovered forming a re-entry circuit. This slow-fast re-entry circuit is found in around 90% of patients with AVNRT.

after the QRS complex (if you're lucky) but more often than not be buried within the QRS complex itself. The circuit arises due to the relative refractoriness of the slow and fast conducting pathways within the AV node itself.

AV re-entry tachycardias may be difficult to differentiate on the surface ECG from junctional tachycardias. Re-entry tachycardias tend to be faster with a 1:1 relationship between the P waves and QRS complexes. These tachycardias are usually associated with structurally normal hearts. Junctional tachycardias also produce retrograde P waves but often there is dissociation of sinus activity with the sporadic appearance of sinus P waves on the ECG. This type of tachycardia is frequently associated with heart disease and digitalis toxicity.

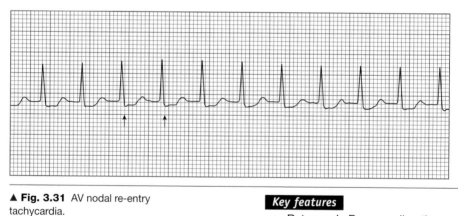

▲ **Fig. 3.31** AV nodal re-entry tachycardia.

Key features

- Retrograde P waves directly after or within QRS complex
- Rate 130–250 bpm

VENTRICULAR RHYTHMS

Ventricular ectopics

Ventricular ectopics arise from an irritable focus within the ventricular myocardium and are unmistakably broad and bizarre-looking. This is because the ventricular impulse is initiated at a point away from the specialised conduction tissue and hence the spread of depolarisation is slower. When a single ectopic focus is active the ectopic beats are described as being "unifocal". When two or more ectopic foci are active the beats are described as "multifocal".

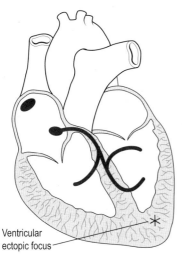

Ventricular
ectopic focus

◀ **Fig. 3.32** Ectopic impulse arising from the ventricular myocardium.

CAUSES

- Caffeine and other stimulants
- Cardiac surgery
- Cardiomyopathy
- Coronary artery disease

- Drug effects (e.g. digoxin or other proarrhythmic drugs)
- Electrolyte disturbances
- Idiopathic
- Myocardial infarction.

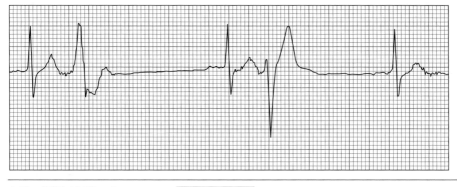

▲ **Fig. 3.33** Multifocal ventricular ectopics arise from multiple foci with varying morphology.

Key features

- Early ventricular beat with no associated P wave
- Broad and bizarre QRS
- Compensatory pause

Different types of ventricular ectopics

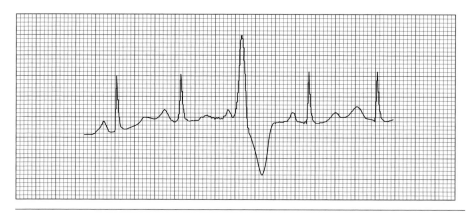

▲ **Fig. 3.34** End-diastolic ventricular ectopic. The ventricular ectopic occurs at the end of diastole following a sinus P wave.

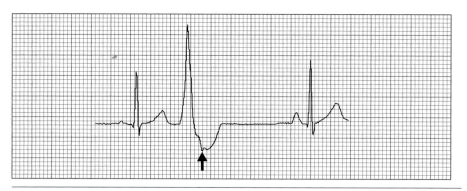

▲ **Fig. 3.35** The ventricular ectopic impulse activates the atria retrogradely causing an inverted P wave to be inscribed on the ectopic T wave.

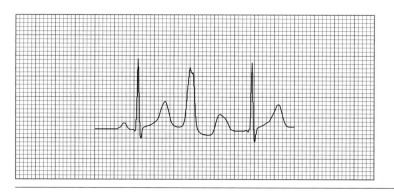

▲ **Fig. 3.36** Interpolated ventricular ectopics occur midway between two normal beats with no compensatory pause.

Quantifying ectopic beats

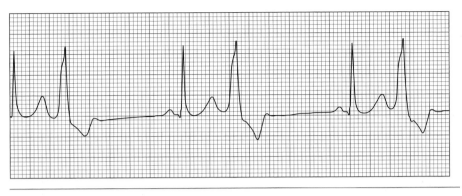

▲ **Fig. 3.37** Ventricular bigeminy One ectopic beat following every one normal beat.

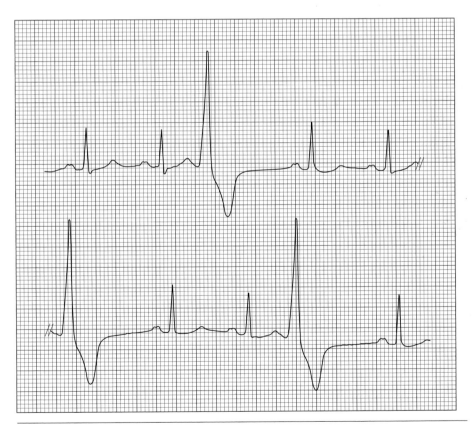

▲ **Fig. 3.38** Ventricular trigeminy. One ectopic beat following every two normal beats. (Note rhythm shown is continuous.)

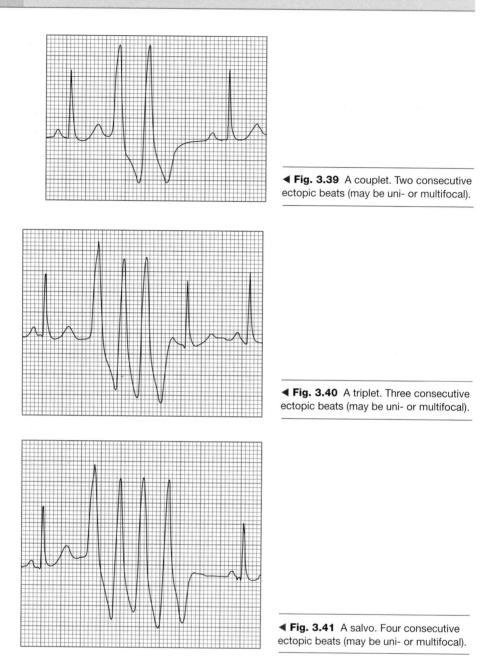

◀ **Fig. 3.39** A couplet. Two consecutive ectopic beats (may be uni- or multifocal).

◀ **Fig. 3.40** A triplet. Three consecutive ectopic beats (may be uni- or multifocal).

◀ **Fig. 3.41** A salvo. Four consecutive ectopic beats (may be uni- or multifocal).

Significance

A few unifocal ventricular ectopics at rest or on exercise is not associated with an increased clinical risk for heart disease. Even frequent ectopics at rest which disappear on exercise have no prognostic significance. However, frequent multifocal ventricular ectopics and increasing numbers of ectopics on exercise are often associated with an increased cardiovascular risk and mortality.

Frequent ventricular ectopic activity (including R-on-T phenomena) after myocardial infarction is common and may not necessarily reflect a higher risk for ventricular fibrillation or cardiac death. Indeed the Cardiac Arrythmia Suppression Trial (1989) showed that the administration of encainide and flecainide (Vaughan-Williams type IC drugs) for asymptomatic or minimally asymptomatic ventricular ectopics after infarction resulted in a higher mortality as compared to placebo. There is, additionally, no strong evidence in favour of the routine use of amiodarone or sotalol. Routine treatment after an MI includes the use of beta-blockers, angiotensin-converting enzymes, statins, omega-3 fatty acids, and, most recently, eplerenone, all of which decrease mortality (including sudden cardiac death) and/or incidence of heart failure.

The presence of frequent ventricular arrhythmias after thrombolysis and revascularisation is a normal occurrence and indicates reperfusion. Indeed they are often called reperfusion arrhythmias and only need treatment if symptomatic, prolonged or extremely frequent.

Monomorphic ventricular tachycardia (VT)

Ventricular tachycardia is often referred to as a broad complex tachycardia. Remember, though, that this term encompasses atrial arrhythmias with broad complex QRS con-

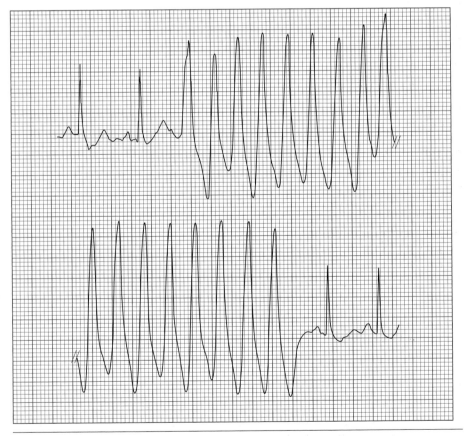

▲ **Fig. 3.42** Monomorphic VT. (Note rhythm shown is continuous.)

Key features
- Broad complex QRS
- QRS is regular
- Rate greater than 120 bpm

duction and does not specifically relate to VT. When you are describing an arrhythmia it is important to be as specific as possible because different rhythms require different treatments. A discussion of the differential diagnosis of these arrhythmias follows this section.

By definition ventricular tachycardia consists of five or more unifocal ventricular ectopics in a row at a rate in excess of 120–140 bpm. This type of tachycardia is sometimes also referred to as "monomorphic" meaning that the site of origin is a single ectopic focus. The ectopic focus can occur from anywhere within the ventricular myocardium. The tachycardia is said to be "sustained" if it lasts for more than 30 seconds.

Causes can be divided as follows.

ACUTE CAUSES

- Acute myocardial infarction
- Cardiac catheterisation
- Electrolyte abnormalities
- Hypothermia
- Idiopathic
- Myocarditis
- Rapid AV conduction in pre-excitation syndromes
- Valvular heart disease.

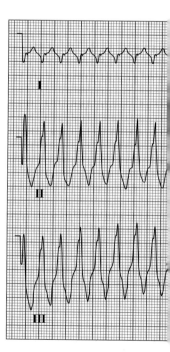

▶ **Fig. 3.43** Right ventricular outflow tract tachycardia.

Key features

- Left bundle branch block pattern
- Right axis deviation

PREDISPOSING CONDITIONS

- Arrhythmogenic right ventricular dysplasia
- Brugada syndrome
- Cardiac surgery
- Cardiomyopathy of any cause (ischaemia, dilated cardiomyopathy, hypertrophic cardiomyopathy, restrictive cardiomyopathy)
- Congenital structural heart disease
- Long QT syndrome
- Mitral valve prolapse
- Valvular heart disease.

While monomorphic ventricular tachycardia is predominantly seen in various forms of heart disease, right ventricular outflow tract (RVOT) tachycardia and fascicular ventricular tachycardia are two types of monomorphic tachycardias associated with structurally normal hearts.

Right ventricular outflow tract tachycardia

A ventricular tachycardia arising in the right ventricular outflow tract will produce a left bundle branch block-type pattern ECG. (Left bundle branch block is described in detail in the Intervals and waveforms section of this chapter.) Also because the impulse is spread inferiorly there is additional right axis deviation.

Often this type of tachycardia is paroxysmal and the patient will present with exertional symptoms. Occasionally, however, the tachycardia may occur at rest in non-sustained repetitive runs. Adenosine may terminate the VT, and beta-blockers and verapamil can suppress recurrence.

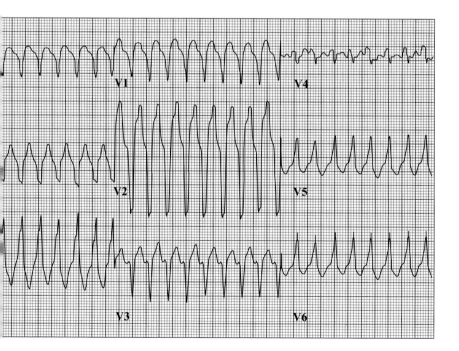

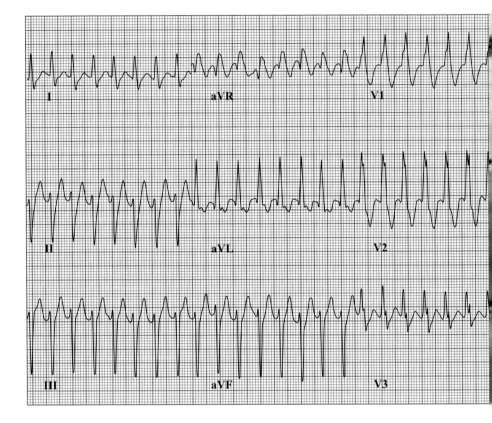

Fascicular tachycardia

This type of tachycardia most commonly arises from the posterior fascicle of the left bundle branch although it may, more rarely, arise from the anterior fascicle. For tachycardias originating from the posterior fascicle a right bundle branch block pattern with left axis deviation is seen on the surface ECG. If the site of origin is the anterior fascicle then a right bundle branch block pattern will develop with a right axis deviation. (Both right bundle branch block and causes of axis deviation are discussed in the Intervals and waveforms section of this chapter.)

Fascicular tachycardia may be treated successfully with verapamil or diltiazem. Both RVOT and fascicular tachycardias can be eliminated by radiofrequency ablation.

Polymorphic ventricular tachycardia

Polymorphic ventricular tachycardia, as the name implies, is the result of rapidly discharging multifocal ventricular ectopics.

Polymorphic ventricular tachycardia is most often seen during acute myocardial infarction or ischaemia and occurs in the presence of a normal QT interval (compare with Torsades de pointes below).

Torsades de pointes

Literally meaning "twisting of points" this is a type of polymorphic ventricular tachycardia seen in the presence of a pre-existing long QT interval. This name stems from the

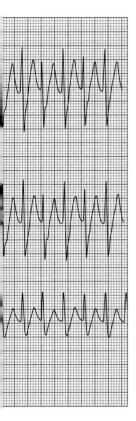

◀ **Fig. 3.44** Posterior fascicular ventricular tachycardia.

Key features

Posterior fascicular tachycardia
- Right bundle branch block
- Left axis deviation

Anterior fascicular tachycardia
- Right bundle branch block
- Right axis deviation

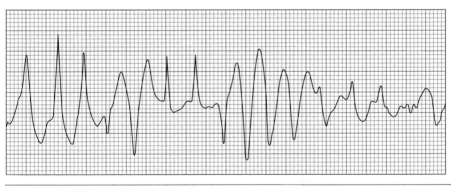

▲ **Fig. 3.45** Polymorphic ventricular tachycardia.

Key features

- Broad QRS with multiple morphologies
- QRS rate greater than 120 bpm

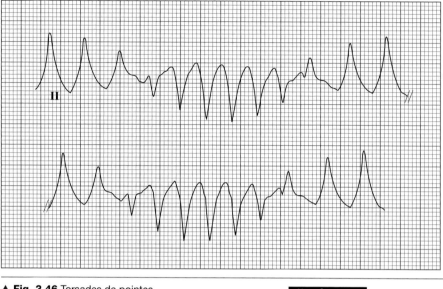

▲ **Fig. 3.46** Torsades de pointes. This ECG was taken from a 55-year-old patient who had been prescribed sotalol for frequent paroxysms of AF. He had been to his GP for treatment of a chest infection three days before he was transported to hospital in a collapsed state. He was pale, sweaty and hypotensive, when he was put on the cardiac monitor. (Note rhythm shown is continuous.)

Key features
- Broad multifocal QRS complexes
- QRS rate greater than 120 bpm

fact that the axis of the resultant QRS vector appears to twist around the isoelectric line.

CAUSES
- Drug effects (e.g. antiarrhythmias and tricyclic antidepressants)
- Hypokalaemia
- Prolonged QT interval.

Accelerated idioventricular rhythm

This is defined as six or more consecutive unifocal ventricular ectopics at a rate of 40–120 bpm. It is often called slow VT (although this is a bit of a misnomer). It is encountered predominantly during acute myocardial infarction and is benign.

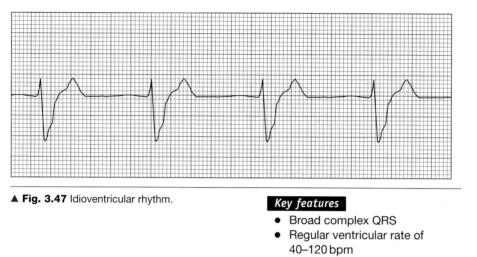

▲ **Fig. 3.47** Idioventricular rhythm.

Key features

- Broad complex QRS
- Regular ventricular rate of 40–120 bpm
- Dissociated atrial activity

Ventricular fibrillation (VF)

This is bad news and if not treated rapidly will result in death. Fortunately VF is a shockable rhythm and can be converted during defibrillation.

CAUSES

- Acute myocardial infarction
- Cardiomyopathy
- Drug toxicity
- Electrocution
- Electrolyte disturbances
- Ischaemic heart disease
- Long QT syndromes.

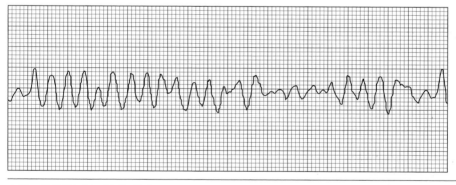

▲ **Fig. 3.48** Ventricular fibrillation.

Key features

- Irregular, chaotic oscillations of the baseline

DIFFERENTIAL DIAGNOSIS OF BROAD COMPLEX TACHYCARDIAS

Perhaps one of the biggest challenges in electrocardiography is the differentiation of broad complex arrhythmias. How do we know, for instance, if the rhythm we are looking at is ventricular in origin or a supraventricular rhythm with an intraventricular block or aberrant conduction? Table 3.5 below lists the various causes of a broad complex QRS. The identification of the origin of broad complex tachyarrhythmias is important because ventricular and supraventricular arrhythmias require different patient management.

The features distinguishing ventricular tachycardia from supraventricular rhythms include:

- Independent atrial activity. Described as the presence of dissociated P waves during VT provided there is normal underlying sinus activity. Note that the atrial rate should be less than the ventricular rate.
- Capture beats. The timing of atrial activity occurring at a particular point in the cycle so that the atria "capture" the ventricles and a normal QRS ensues within a run of VT.
- Fusion beats. When a captured beat occurs simultaneously with a ventricular ectopic beat and the two "collide" – the result is a combination of the two.
- Concordance. Concordance throughout the chest leads (V1–V6) is diagnostic for VT. Concordance means that all QRS complexes are pointing in the same direction. It is described as being either positive (with upright complexes) or negative (downward complexes). But beware! Positive concordance may also be seen in patients with Wolf–Parkinson–White syndrome type A.

Isolated ventricular ectopics leading up to or following a run of broad complex tachycardia should also provide clues as to its origin. If the QRS complex morphology during the tachycardia matches that of the ventricular ectopic beats then the diagnosis of VT is more certain. A cautionary note is required here because it is important that what you are comparing are, indeed, ventricular ectopics and not aberrantly conducted atrial

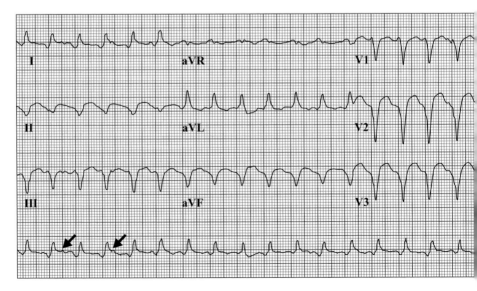

Table 3.5 Causes of broad complex QRS

Ventricular ectopy	Intraventricular block	Aberrant conduction
Ventricular ectopic beats	Right bundle branch block	Short coupling interval
Ventricular tachycardia	Left bundle branch block	Ashman's phenomenon
Ventricular/idioventricular escape beats or rhythms	Non-specific intraventricular conduction delay	
Ventricular fibrillation		

ectopics! The presence of either a premature or abnormally-shaped P wave, if visualised, should give the game away.

Extremely bizarre QRS complexes which fit no intraventricular block pattern are strongly suggestive of ventricular ectopy and are especially common in the elderly, in patients with a history of cardiac disease and in the case of digitalis toxicity. The absence of Ashman's phenomenon is also a clue (see below).

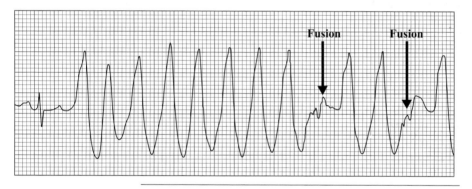

▲ **Fig. 3.49a** The presence of fusion beats is consistent with ventricular tachycardia.

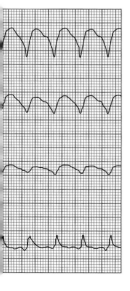

◄ **Fig. 3.49b** This ECG shows negative concordance throughout the precordial leads. Dissociated P waves (arrowed) are seen in the initial portion of the rhythm strip. Additionally there is left axis deviation. The ECG was taken from a 25-year-old professional basketball player who was hospitalised after an episode of loss of consciousness during a game. His father and paternal uncle had both died suddenly before the age of forty. A recent cardiological check-up had revealed normal clinical, electrocardiographic and echocardiographic findings. He was conscious when this ECG was recorded, but was feeling light-headed and nauseous. The findings are consistent with ventricular tachycardia.

The width of the QRS complex may also hold clues. A QRS width of greater than 0.14 secs with right bundle branch block or 0.16 secs with left bundle branch block patterns favours VT.

Finally, if you are fortunate enough to witness the end of a run of tachycardia closer inspection of the post-tachycardia pause may also offer some clues. VT is always followed by a post-tachycardia pause whereas supraventricular tachycardias often are not (this is particularly true for atrial fibrillation).

Atrial or AV junctional tachycardias with broad complex QRS conduction
These rhythms may be identified by any of the following:

- Premature or abnormal morphology P waves associated with the QRS
- The presence of an initial short coupling interval or Ashman's phenomenon
- No long pause following ectopic beats or run of tachycardia
- Grossly irregular R–R intervals
- Pre-existing intraventricular block on previous ECGs.

Aberrant conduction
Aberrant conduction in this context relates specifically to the occurrence of an *intermittent* broad complex beat or rhythm that is supraventricular in origin. It may therefore be a feature of any supraventricular rhythm. The term is not used, however, in the presence of pre-existing right or left bundle branch block.

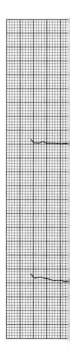

▶ **Fig. 3.50** Sinus rhythm with frequent supraventricular ectopics demonstrating the coupling interval.

What causes aberrant conduction?

Aberrant ventricular conduction arises when a supraventricular impulse is conducted to the ventricles at a time when one of the bundle branches is still refractory. This happens either due to a short coupling interval or secondary to something called Ashman's phenomenon. Both are described below. The QRS configuration of the conducted impulse is typically that of right bundle branch block (in up to 85% of cases). Less often a left bundle branch block pattern is seen. Occasionally the ECG may show alternating right and left bundle branch block patterns in the same patient. Anterior or posterior hemiblock configurations may also be seen if either one of the fascicles of the left bundle branch is refractory at the time of conduction. If both bundle branches are equally refractory the impulse will be completely non-conducted, as in the case of non-conducted supraventricular ectopics.

Short coupling interval

The coupling interval is the time between a normal beat and the ectopic beat that follows it. The earlier the supraventricular ectopic beat occurs, the more likely it is to fall into the partial refractory period of the ventricular cycle and the higher the chance, therefore, of the ectopic beat being aberrantly conducted.

Ashman's phenomenon

Ashman's phenomenon, first described in 1945, may be seen in any cardiac rhythm as a result of a prolonged ventricular cycle. Hence aberrant conduction may be due to slow, as well as fast, heart rhythms. It is often seen in arrhythmias such as multifocal atrial tachycardia or atrial fibrillation due to the irregular R–R intervals where a prolonged ventricular cycle is frequently followed by a much shorter cycle which initiates an aberrantly conducted beat.

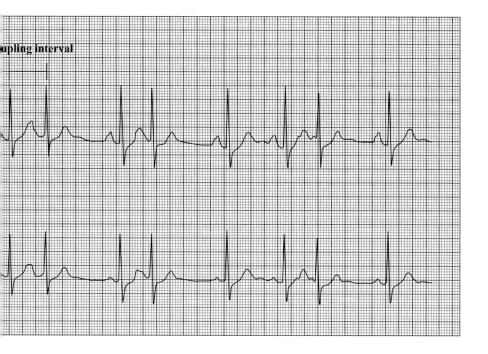

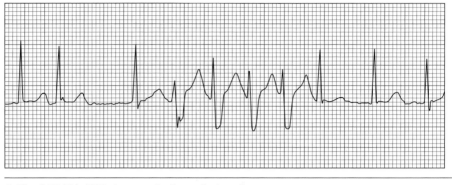

▲ **Fig. 3.51** This ECG shows a short run of a broad complex tachyarrhythmia during a period of atrial fibrillation. Note that the first broadly-conducted beat follows a short, then long, ventricular cycle. There is no compensatory pause following the fourth broad beat. This finding is consistent with aberrantly conducted AF.

The mechanism is the same for isolated aberrantly conducted beats as well as for consecutively occurring aberrancy (as shown).

The broad QRS complex is a functional finding because it is said that the longer the ventricular cycle the longer the refractory period following it. An early beat following a long R–R interval will therefore encounter a bundle branch system which is still partially refractory.

A general approach to broad complex tachycardias

Step 1: Cardiovascular stability

Cardiovascular instability (heart failure, hypotension, shock) occurs in both ventricular and supraventricular arrhythmias, but slightly favours a ventricular origin.

Step 2: History and old ECGs (if possible!)

The presence of the same QRS morphology during sinus rhythm confirms a supraventricular origin.

A history of severe myocardial disease (IHD, cardiomyopathy, congenital heart disease, heart failure, family history of sudden cardiac death, cardiotoxic drugs) is somewhat more suggestive of ventricular origin. A long post-tachycardia compensatory pause on a strip of ECG obtained during a temporary reversion to sinus rhythm indicates VT.

Step 3: Rate and rhythm

Because of the overlap of heart rate ranges during a tachycardia, heart rate assessment can provide only limited clues. Both ventricular and supraventricular tachycardia may produce heart rates in the region of 120–180 bpm. However, in ventricular tachycardia the heart rate seldom exceeds 200 bpm and at a rate of 150 bpm you should certainly consider the possibility of atrial flutter with 2:1 block. Heart rates of 230 bpm and above strongly suggest pre-excited AF.

It is very unusual for VT to appear irregular whereas it is not unusual for atrial tachycardias to appear irregular, particularly in the initial portion of the arrhythmia. Atrial fibrillation will always look "irregularly irregular". Additionally look for the presence of flutter waves.

Step 4: "Traditional" criteria:

- Dissociated P waves
- Fusion and capture beats
- Concordance
- QRS > 0.14 s
- Left axis deviation.

All favour VT. Unfortunately, these easily accessible criteria are helpful in only about 30% of cases.

Step 5: The expert's trick-of-the-trade

Do not be too concerned by the apparent complexity of the notes below. Everyone finds them hard to memorise at first. Unfortunately there's no easy solution: if you want to use them, you have to commit them to memory. The more you apply these criteria, the better you will become.

Firstly, decide if the ECG resembles a RBBB or LBBB pattern. If RBBB, ask yourself (a) is the second R wave in V1 (the R') larger than the first R wave? And (b) is the R wave in V6 of larger amplitude than the ensuing S wave? If the answer to one or both of these questions is yes, think SVT. If the answer is no, think VT. A monophasic R, a qR, or an RS in V1 is also suggestive of VT.

If LBBB, ask yourself – is the delay between the onset of the QRS and the nadir of the S wave (the lowermost point of the S wave) in V1 less than 70 ms (almost two small squares)? If yes, then think SVT. If no, think VT. Also, a Q wave in V6 suggests VT, and an R wave but no Q wave in V6 suggests SVT.

Despite all of the above you may still get ECGs that defy classification. Experience is always an asset, and far more important than any theoretical background. This is why an early expert opinion is the best way forward in many cases.

CARDIAC ARREST RHYTHMS

There are four heart rhythms associated with cardiac arrest. These are:

- Ventricular fibrillation
- Ventricular tachycardia (pulseless) } "shockable"
- Asystole
- Pulseless electrical activity (PEA). } "non-shockable"

The so-called "shockable" rhythms should be treated with prompt defibrillation and are associated with a more favourable outcome. For non-shockable rhythms (sometimes called "non-VF/VT" rhythms) the outcome is less favourable unless a reversible cause can be found and treated. Reversible causes of cardiac arrest are listed below.

- Hypoxia
- Hypovolaemia
- Hypo/hyperkalaemia (and other metabolic disorders)
- Hypothermia
- Tension pneumothorax
- Tamponade
- Toxic/therapeutic disorders
- Thrombo-embolic and mechanical obstruction.

Adapted from the European Resuscitation Council Guidelines for Adult Advanced Life Support (2000).

Ventricular fibrillation

Ventricular fibrillation is by far the most common rhythm at the time of cardiac arrest and should be treated with prompt defibrillation because the chance of successful defibrillation declines by 7–10% for each minute the rhythm persists. If defibrillation is not immediately possible then basic life support should be commenced until a defibrillator can be found.

Check!

Fine VF on an ECG monitor may look like asystole. *Check your ECG gains.* VF is a shockable rhythm. Asystole is not.

Ventricular tachycardia

Ventricular tachycardia in a patient who is not haemodynamically compromised may be well tolerated. However pulseless VT is clearly not compatible with life. Again, prompt defibrillation is required.

If a defibrillator is not readily available and the arrest is witnessed it may be possible (within the first 30 seconds) to convert either pulseless VT or VF back to a perfusing rhythm with a precordial thump. A precordial thump is a sharp blow with a closed fist to the patient's sternum.

Asystole

Literally meaning "without systole", the asystolic heart demonstrates no electrical output represented by a flat line on the ECG. Cardiopulmonary resuscitation (CPR) should be commenced without delay.

For a diagnosis of asystole to be made it is important to first check that the ECG leads are all connected and connected correctly. As previously mentioned the ECG gain should also be checked to ensure that the rhythm is not fine VF. It is also important to watch closely throughout resuscitation for the presence of P waves or slow ventricular activity which will require cardiac pacing.

Check!

Spurious asystole may follow defibrillation due to "myocardial stunning". CPR should be commenced for one minute and the rhythm and pulse rechecked before asystole is diagnosed.

Pulseless electrical activity (PEA)

Also known as electromechanical dissociation (EMD), this exhibits the paradox of an ECG rhythm compatible with life in a patient in cardiac arrest. PEA therefore serves to

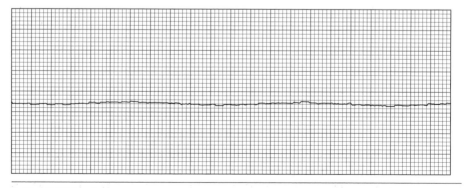

▲ **Fig. 3.52** Asystole.

remind us of the adage: treat the patient, not the trace.

Treatment for PEA is the same as for asystole with identification and correction of any potentially reversible cause.

Check!

What's the rate? A PEA of less than 60 bpm can be treated with atropine.

PERI-ARREST ARRHYTHMIAS

Peri-arrest arrhythmias may pretty much be any cardiac arrhythmia which results in an inappropriate haemodynamic state for the patient and which may, potentially, lead to cardiac arrest.

These arrhythmias may broadly be defined as:
- Bradycardias
- Broad complex tachycardias and
- Narrow complex tachycardias.

The treatment of these arrhythmias is dependent on adverse clinical signs or the risk of potential complications. All of the following arrhythmias are described in more detail in the sections above. Adverse clinical signs are listed only to demonstrate when intervention is necessary based on ECG findings.

Bradycardia

In the context of peri-arrest, bradycardia is defined as a heart rate of less than 40 bpm. In practice the rate is less important if the patient is symptomatic.

Adverse signs
- Systolic blood pressure of less than 90 mmHg
- Ventricular arrhythmias
- Heart failure.

Associated risk factors for asystole
- Recent asystole
- Mobitz type II AV block
- Complete heart block
- Ventricular pauses (greater than 3 seconds).

Broad complex tachycardia

For the arrest and peri-arrest scenario aberrantly conducted supraventricular tachycardias are assumed to be ventricular in origin. Again, the rate of the tachycardia is less important than how the patient is feeling but rates above 150 bpm are considered, in this context, to be more ominous.

Adverse signs
- Systolic blood pressure less than 90 mmHg
- Chest pain
- Heart failure
- Heart rate greater than 150 bpm.

For patients with a broad complex tachycardia and no pulse you should follow the cardiac arrest algorithm for VF/pulseless VT. If a pulse is present but the patient displays adverse signs, cardioversion is indicated and expert help should be sought. In the absence of adverse signs when broad complex tachycardias are well tolerated by the patient, antiarrhythmic therapy should be initiated. At this point you should start to consider if the tachycardia is ventricular or supraventricular in origin (see discussion above).

Narrow complex tachycardia

Any supraventricular tachycardia causing haemodynamic compromise should be treated with cardioversion. Generally, supraventricular tachycardias with rates less than 200 bpm are better tolerated. Under these circumstances vagal manoeuvres or anti-arrhythmic therapy is the first line choice of treatment. Vagal manoeuvres include the Valsalva manoeuvre (forced expiration against a closed glottis), eyeball pressure and carotid sinus massage.

Adverse signs
- Systolic BP less than 90 mmHg
- Chest pain
- Heart failure
- Heart rate greater than 200 bpm.

Patients presenting with atrial fibrillation are additionally classified according to their level of risk. High-risk patients should be treated as for other problematic supraventricular tachycardias with cardioversion. For patients with slow AF the bradycardia treatment options apply.

High risk
- Heart rate greater than 150 bpm
- Chest pain
- Critical perfusion.

Intermediate risk
- Heart rate 100–150 bpm
- Breathlessness
- Poor perfusion.

Low risk
- Heart rate less than 100 bpm
- Mild or no symptoms
- Good perfusion.

PACEMAKER RHYTHMS

Before pacemaker rhythms are described it is necessary to first provide some background.

Indications for pacing

Pacemakers are used predominantly in the treatment of slow heart rhythms. The use of pacemakers in the treatment of fast heart rhythms (antitachycardia devices for atrial arrhythmias) is a more recent innovation. Implantable cardiovertor-defibrillators (ICDs) are used in the treatment of ventricular tachyarrhythmias including ventricular tachycardia and fibrillation (see below).

The indications for pacing are based on both the resting ECG findings and on patient symptoms.

- Complete (third degree) heart block in patients with a history of syncope or pre-syncope. Pacing should also be considered in asymptomatic, awake, patients with a ventricular rate of less than 40 bpm or with pauses of greater than three seconds because of the risk of asystole. Asymptomatic patients with congenital complete heart block do not usually require pacing.
- Mobitz type I second degree AV block requires pacing only in symptomatic individuals. Mobitz type II, regardless of symptoms, requires pacing because of the risk of progression to complete AV block.
- Sick sinus syndrome in patients with symptomatic bradycardia.
- Bifascicular and trifascicular block do not usually require pacing unless there is a history of syncope or evidence of higher degrees of block.
- Chronic atrial fibrillation following AV node ablation.
- Hypersensitive carotid sinus syndrome.

Pacing modes

Pacemaker modes are assigned generic codes as defined by the North American Society for Pacing and Electrophysiology (NASPE) and by the British Pacing and Elec-trophysiology Group (BPEG) which are based on the type of pacing system implanted.

Pacing modes are depicted by three or four letters as shown in Table 3.6 below. For antitachyarrhythmia devices an additional, fifth, letter is also added.

The most common pacing rhythms you are likely to encounter are as follows.

Table 3.6 Pacing mode abbreviations

I	II	III	IV	V
Chamber(s) paced	Chamber(s) sensed	Response to sensing	Programmability/ Rate modulation	Antitachycardia functions
O	O	O	O	O
A	A	T	P	P
V	V	I	M	S
D	D	D	C	D
			R	

O = none; A = atrium; V = ventricle; D = dual; T = triggered; I = inhibited; P = single programmable (with specific respect to programmability); M = multiprogrammable; C = communicating; R = rate modulation; P = pacing (with specific respect to antitachyarrhythmia devices); S = shock; D = dual (pace and shock – with specific respect to antitachyarrhythmia devices).

AAI

This is a single chamber system in which the atrium is paced and sensed. The pacemaker will be inhibited (that is, it will not pace) if it sees the heart's intrinsic activity. This is not as frequently used as it once was and is typically restricted to patients with disorders affecting only the sinus node in whom the AV node is unaffected. An additional letter is often added so that the pacemaker may respond to the physical demands of the patient by increasing the rate of pacing (AAIR). This is a feature of rate responsive pacing.

Conduction through the ventricles is via the normal conduction system hence the QRS complex is typically narrow (in the absence of pre-existing bundle branch block).

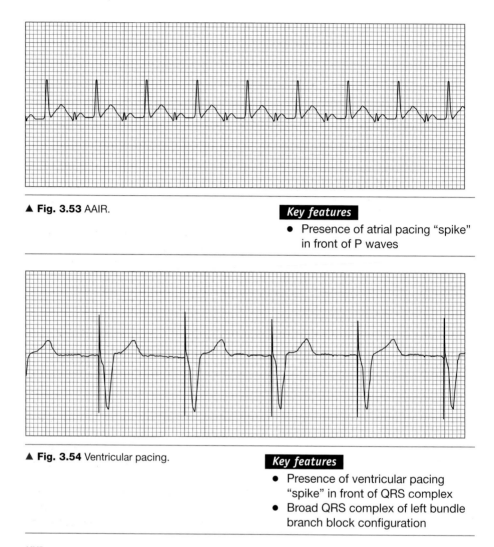

▲ **Fig. 3.53** AAIR.

Key features

- Presence of atrial pacing "spike" in front of P waves

▲ **Fig. 3.54** Ventricular pacing.

Key features

- Presence of ventricular pacing "spike" in front of QRS complex
- Broad QRS complex of left bundle branch block configuration

VVI

This, again, is a single chamber pacing system wherein the chamber paced and sensed is the right ventricle and the response to sensing is inhibition of pacing. This is still widely used, with or without the addition of rate responsiveness (VVIR) in patients with chronic atrial fibrillation.

The QRS complex is broad because depolarisation of the ventricles has been initiated by the pacing lead placed at the apex of the right ventricle away from the normal conduction system. Because of this, ventricular pacing produces a left bundle branch block pattern on the ECG.

DDD

Dual chamber devices are more commonly selected with or without the addition of rate responsive pacing depending on the needs of the patient (DDDR). In dual chamber systems, pacing and sensing occurs in both the atrium and ventricle. In the DDD system a sensed event will either inhibit the pacemaker or trigger the pacemaker into a timing cycle whereby the atrium and ventricle are paced in synchrony.

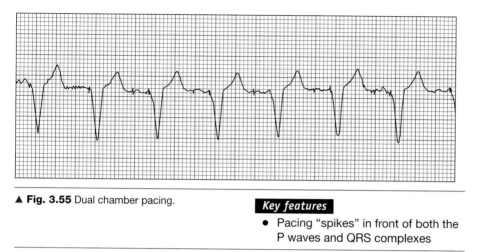

▲ **Fig. 3.55** Dual chamber pacing.

Key features

- Pacing "spikes" in front of both the P waves and QRS complexes

Upper rate behaviour

The ability of a pacemaker to sense in the atrium and then pace in the ventricle is a feature unique to dual chamber systems. This is all well and good during periods of normal atrial activity but what happens to the ventricular rate in the event of a supra-ventricular tachycardia such as atrial flutter or atrial tachycardia? Pacemakers clearly need a mechanism for dealing with high atrial rates so that a dangerously rapid ventricular response does not develop. This mechanism is referred to as the pacemaker's upper rate limit (or maximum tracking rate) and this refers to the maximum rate at which the pacemaker will pace in the ventricle in response to sensed atrial activity.

Atrial activity occurring at rates above the upper rate limit will produce, on the surface ECG, a rhythm similar to Wenckebach's phenomenon with the intermittent presence of P waves which are not conducted to the ventricles.

Excessively high atrial rates, as seen in the case of atrial fibrillation, will cause the pacemaker to switch pacing modes (so-called "mode-switch" episodes) to a non-atrial tracking mode such as VVI. The upper tracking rate on most pacemakers is usually set around 120–130 bpm.

Pacing problems detectable on the surface ECG

Undersensing

Failure to sense the heart's intrinsic activity will result in pacing which on the surface ECG will appear inappropriate. This is caused by two main problems: inappropriate programmed settings or secondary to problems with the pacing lead such as lead tip fibrosis or dislodgement.

CAUSES

- Inappropriate programming
- Lead tip fibrosis or dislodgement.

Oversensing

Oversensing results in pacemaker inhibition and occurs when the pacemaker sees signals from other sources which it misinterprets as the heart's own intrinsic activity.

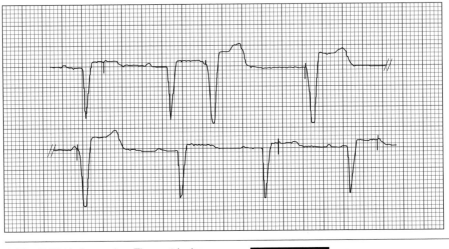

▲ **Fig. 3.56** Undersensing. The ventricular pacing spikes are discharged at 60 bpm even though this patient has intrinsic ventricular activity with some spikes seen falling upon the T wave of the preceding beats. (Note that the rhythm shown is continuous.)

Key features

- Pacing spikes occur at the pacemakers programmed lower rate limit and appear to occur irrespective of the patient's own intrinsic rhythm

These other sources may be myopotentials, electromagnetic interference and, sometimes, even intrinsic T waves. Another potential cause of oversensing, particularly in older devices, is crosstalk. Crosstalk occurs in dual chamber pacing when one of the pacing leads "sees" activity in the other chamber. In the case of the ventricular lead, atrial activity is sensed and misinterpreted as an intrinsic R wave. This has the disastrous result of inhibiting ventricular output which, in the pacing-dependent patient, leads to ventricular standstill.

You should suspect oversensing in the following circumstances:

- The surface ECG shows the patient's own heart rhythm is present and the patient is bradycardic (note that the bradycardia must be at a rate lower than the pacemaker's programmed lower rate limit including any programmed hysteresis*)
- The pacemaker appears to be pacing at a rate lower than the programmed lower rate limit
- The patient presents with an ECG which is the same as at pre-implant
- The patient reports a reoccurrence of symptoms.

Oversensing is remedied by either reprogramming the pacemaker or by removing the source of interference.

Failure to capture

This is seen on the surface ECG as pacing spikes which are not followed by depolarisation.

*Hysteresis is a programmable pacemaker function that allows the patient's own heart rhythm to fall, say 10 bpm, below the lower rate limit of the pacemaker in order to encourage the heart's own intrinsic activity. For instance, in a patient with a pacemaker programmed at a lower rate limit of 60 bpm, the pacemaker will allow the patient's own heart rate to fall as low as 50 bpm before it starts pacing.

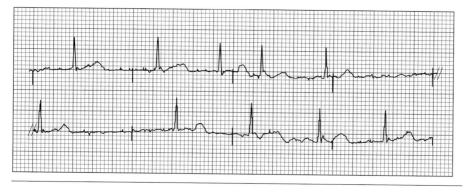

▲ **Fig. 3.57** This ECG shows pacing spikes occurring at the pacemaker's lower rate limits of 60 bpm in spite of the presence of intrinsic rhythm (failure to sense) but also none of the spikes manage to cause the ventricles to depolarise (failure to capture). (Note that the rhythm shown is continuous.)

CAUSES

- Cardiac perforation
- Increased threshold
- Inappropriate programming
- Lead fracture or dislodgement
- Pacemaker battery failure.

Pacemaker-mediated tachycardia (PMT)

A pacemaker-mediated tachycardia may be precipitated by any pacemaker that is capable of sensing in the atrium and pacing in the ventricle and is a well-recognised complication of dual chamber systems.

This so-called "endless loop" tachycardia is initiated due to the presence of retrograde V–A (ventricle-to-atrium) conduction following a ventricular paced event as follows:

> Pacing occurs in the ventricle
> Impulse is conducted retrogradely from ventricle to atrium
> Atrium contracts
> P wave is sensed in the atrium

The ventricular pacing rate, prompted by repeated sensing in the atrium, becomes accelerated up to the pacemaker's maximum tracking rate (see above). Hence, if a patient presents with a tachycardia which is almost exactly at this rate a PMT should be suspected.

Termination may be achieved by any one of the following methods:

- Application of a magnet (stops atrial sensing)
- Reprogramming the pacemaker to a "non-tracking" mode such as VVI or DDI so that sensed P waves do not prompt ventricular pacing
- Extending the pacemaker's atrial refractory period by reprogramming.

Note that not all patients have V–A conduction. However, it is possible that even patients   91

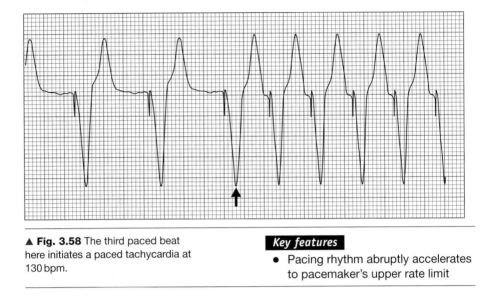

▲ Fig. 3.58 The third paced beat here initiates a paced tachycardia at 130 bpm.

Key features
- Pacing rhythm abruptly accelerates to pacemaker's upper rate limit

presenting with complete AV block may be capable of retrograde AV conduction. Testing for V–A conduction can be carried out pre-implant but is seldom practised.

IMPLANTABLE CARDIOVERTOR-DEFIBRILLATORS (ICDS)

ICDs behave like a normal pacing system in terms of the ability to both pace and sense and so the ECG produced by such a system may resemble any of the pacing rhythms already described above. However, these devices offer a few important additional functions not seen in normal pacemakers.

Antitachycardia pacing
This is usually indicated as a first-line treatment in patients with ventricular tachycardia at a rate of under 180 bpm. Many such episodes are amenable to this technique (also known as overdrive pacing). The onset of a ventricular tachycardia will prompt the device to discharge a "burst" of up to 15 pacing impulses delivered at a rapid rate. If termination of the tachycardia is not achieved after a certain programmed number of pacing attempts low-energy cardioversion may be initiated.

Low-energy cardioversion
This is used either as a back-up to antitachycardia pacing therapy or as a first line option in ventricular tachycardias in excess of 180 bpm. The cardioversion is synchronised with the sensed R wave and the amount of energy delivered may be in the region of between 0.1–34 joules. If cardioversion fails after a preset number of attempts or if the tachycardia accelerates defibrillation may follow.

Defibrillation
This is used for ventricular tachycardias exceeding 180 bpm not amenable to cardioversion or as a first line therapy in ventricular fibrillation. The energy delivered is, again, in the range 0.1–34 joules.

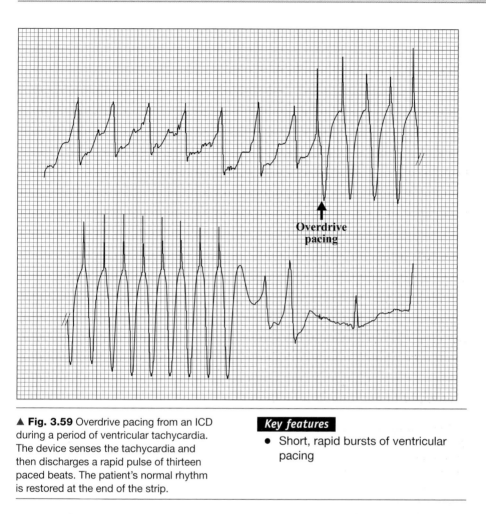

▲ **Fig. 3.59** Overdrive pacing from an ICD during a period of ventricular tachycardia. The device senses the tachycardia and then discharges a rapid pulse of thirteen paced beats. The patient's normal rhythm is restored at the end of the strip.

Key features

- Short, rapid bursts of ventricular pacing

Following successful cardioversion/defibrillation the ICD will return to basic pacing mode as it is known that about 10% of patients will be shocked back into a marked sinus bradycardia.

Inappropriate function

Because ICDs work in a similar way to pacemakers in terms of their sensing abilities, they are also susceptible to similar problems. Oversensing in an ICD may lead to inappropriate pacing or shocking of the patient which may, itself, lead to either VT or VF. In this instance the ICD may be temporarily deactivated by placement of a magnet over the device. You should note that removing the magnet will reactivate the ICD and further shocks may occur. Therefore the magnet should be taped in place until a programmer can be obtained and the device can be programmed off. The application of the magnet will not affect the back-up bradycardia pacing functions.

3.2
Intervals and waveforms: Flowcharts

P WAVES

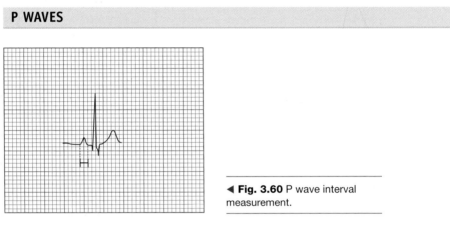

◀ **Fig. 3.60** P wave interval measurement.

Normal values: *Amplitude = 2.5 mm (or 2.5 small squares) high*
                             Duration = 0.08 secs (or 2 small squares) wide

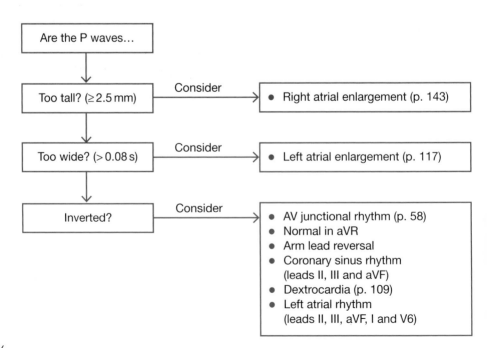

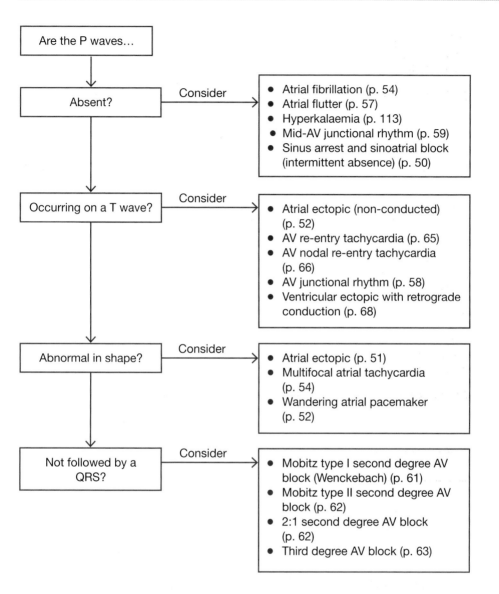

Are the P waves...

Absent? — Consider →
- Atrial fibrillation (p. 54)
- Atrial flutter (p. 57)
- Hyperkalaemia (p. 113)
- Mid-AV junctional rhythm (p. 59)
- Sinus arrest and sinoatrial block (intermittent absence) (p. 50)

Occurring on a T wave? — Consider →
- Atrial ectopic (non-conducted) (p. 52)
- AV re-entry tachycardia (p. 65)
- AV nodal re-entry tachycardia (p. 66)
- AV junctional rhythm (p. 58)
- Ventricular ectopic with retrograde conduction (p. 68)

Abnormal in shape? — Consider →
- Atrial ectopic (p. 51)
- Multifocal atrial tachycardia (p. 54)
- Wandering atrial pacemaker (p. 52)

Not followed by a QRS? — Consider →
- Mobitz type I second degree AV block (Wenckebach) (p. 61)
- Mobitz type II second degree AV block (p. 62)
- 2:1 second degree AV block (p. 62)
- Third degree AV block (p. 63)

THE PR INTERVAL

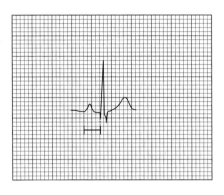

◀ **Fig. 3.61** PR interval measurement.

Normal range
0.12–0.20 secs (3–5 small squares) long

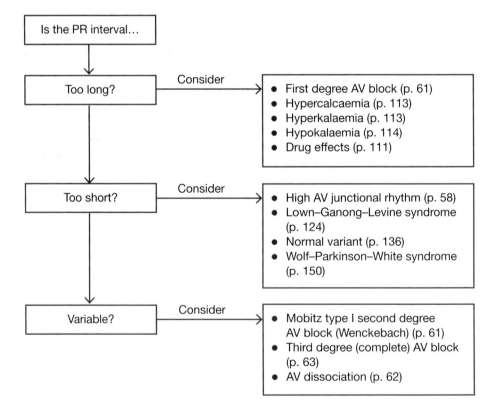

Is the PR interval…

Too long? — Consider →
- First degree AV block (p. 61)
- Hypercalcaemia (p. 113)
- Hyperkalaemia (p. 113)
- Hypokalaemia (p. 114)
- Drug effects (p. 111)

Too short? — Consider →
- High AV junctional rhythm (p. 58)
- Lown–Ganong–Levine syndrome (p. 124)
- Normal variant (p. 136)
- Wolf–Parkinson–White syndrome (p. 150)

Variable? — Consider →
- Mobitz type I second degree AV block (Wenckebach) (p. 61)
- Third degree (complete) AV block (p. 63)
- AV dissociation (p. 62)

Q WAVES

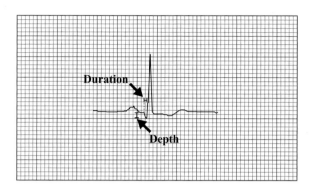

◀ **Fig. 3.62** Q wave depth and duration measurements.

Normal range
Less than 2 mm (2 small squares) deep
Represent less than 25% of the height of the associated R wave
Less than 0.04 secs (1 small square) wide

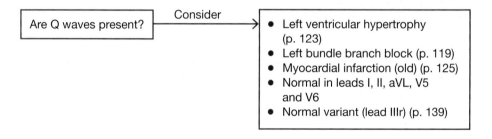

Are Q waves present? ──Consider──→
- Left ventricular hypertrophy (p. 123)
- Left bundle branch block (p. 119)
- Myocardial infarction (old) (p. 125)
- Normal in leads I, II, aVL, V5 and V6
- Normal variant (lead IIIr) (p. 139)

THE QRS COMPLEX

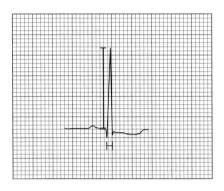

◀ **Fig. 3.63** QRS duration and amplitude measurements.

Normal range
R and S wave amplitude no greater than 25 mm (5 large squares)
Complex width no greater than 0.10 secs (2.5 small squares)

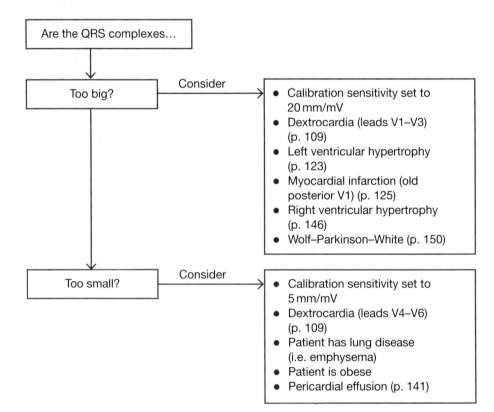

Are the QRS complexes...

Too big?   Consider →
- Calibration sensitivity set to 20 mm/mV
- Dextrocardia (leads V1–V3) (p. 109)
- Left ventricular hypertrophy (p. 123)
- Myocardial infarction (old posterior V1) (p. 125)
- Right ventricular hypertrophy (p. 146)
- Wolf–Parkinson–White (p. 150)

Too small?   Consider →
- Calibration sensitivity set to 5 mm/mV
- Dextrocardia (leads V4–V6) (p. 109)
- Patient has lung disease (i.e. emphysema)
- Patient is obese
- Pericardial effusion (p. 141)

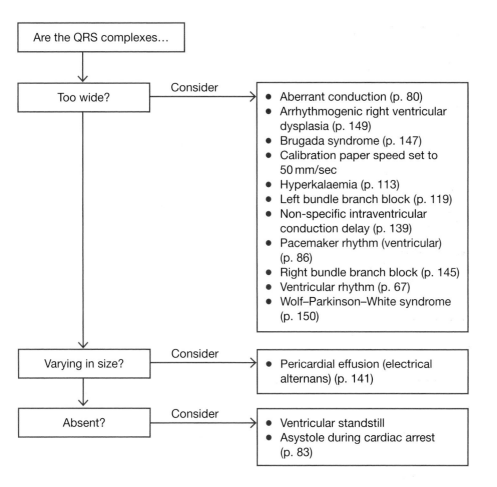

Are the QRS complexes…

Too wide? — Consider →
- Aberrant conduction (p. 80)
- Arrhythmogenic right ventricular dysplasia (p. 149)
- Brugada syndrome (p. 147)
- Calibration paper speed set to 50 mm/sec
- Hyperkalaemia (p. 113)
- Left bundle branch block (p. 119)
- Non-specific intraventricular conduction delay (p. 139)
- Pacemaker rhythm (ventricular) (p. 86)
- Right bundle branch block (p. 145)
- Ventricular rhythm (p. 67)
- Wolf–Parkinson–White syndrome (p. 150)

Varying in size? — Consider →
- Pericardial effusion (electrical alternans) (p. 141)

Absent? — Consider →
- Ventricular standstill
- Asystole during cardiac arrest (p. 83)

THE QT INTERVAL

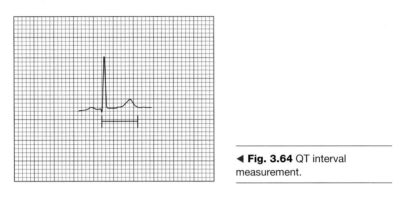

◀ **Fig. 3.64** QT interval measurement.

Normal range
0.35–0.43 secs (approximately 8–11 small squares)

The QT interval should be corrected for heart rate using the following equation:

$$\text{Corrected QT (QTc)} = QT/\sqrt{RR}$$

Where,
QT = the measured QT (in seconds)
RR = the measured R–R interval (in seconds).

Note that most modern ECG machines will do this for you.

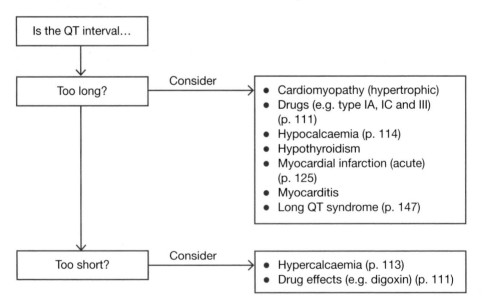

Is the QT interval…

Too long? — Consider →
- Cardiomyopathy (hypertrophic)
- Drugs (e.g. type IA, IC and III) (p. 111)
- Hypocalcaemia (p. 114)
- Hypothyroidism
- Myocardial infarction (acute) (p. 125)
- Myocarditis
- Long QT syndrome (p. 147)

Too short? — Consider →
- Hypercalcaemia (p. 113)
- Drug effects (e.g. digoxin) (p. 111)

THE ST SEGMENT

Normally isoelectric
Elevated = above the isoelectric line
Depressed = below the isoelectric line

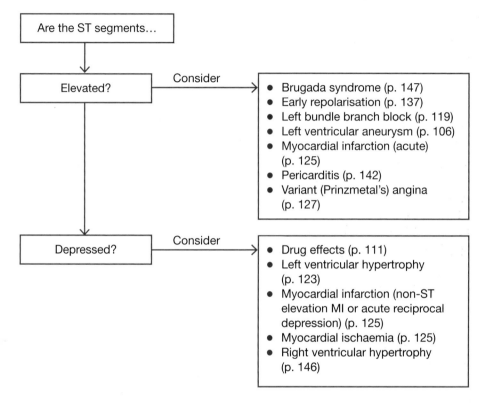

Are the ST segments…

Elevated? — Consider →
- Brugada syndrome (p. 147)
- Early repolarisation (p. 137)
- Left bundle branch block (p. 119)
- Left ventricular aneurysm (p. 106)
- Myocardial infarction (acute) (p. 125)
- Pericarditis (p. 142)
- Variant (Prinzmetal's) angina (p. 127)

Depressed? — Consider →
- Drug effects (p. 111)
- Left ventricular hypertrophy (p. 123)
- Myocardial infarction (non-ST elevation MI or acute reciprocal depression) (p. 125)
- Myocardial ischaemia (p. 125)
- Right ventricular hypertrophy (p. 146)

T WAVES

Normal
Less than two-thirds the height of the associated R wave
Peak is in the same direction as the R wave

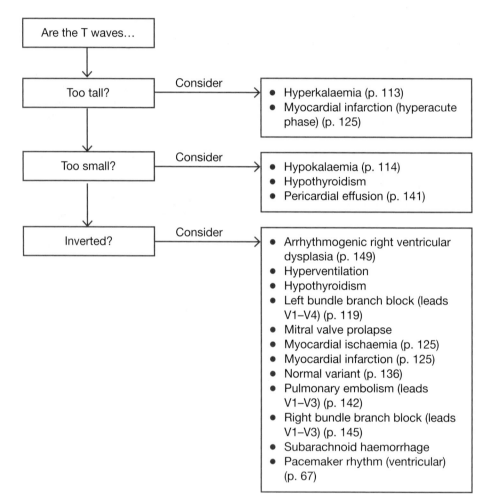

Are the T waves...

Too tall? — Consider →
- Hyperkalaemia (p. 113)
- Myocardial infarction (hyperacute phase) (p. 125)

Too small? — Consider →
- Hypokalaemia (p. 114)
- Hypothyroidism
- Pericardial effusion (p. 141)

Inverted? — Consider →
- Arrhythmogenic right ventricular dysplasia (p. 149)
- Hyperventilation
- Hypothyroidism
- Left bundle branch block (leads V1–V4) (p. 119)
- Mitral valve prolapse
- Myocardial ischaemia (p. 125)
- Myocardial infarction (p. 125)
- Normal variant (p. 136)
- Pulmonary embolism (leads V1–V3) (p. 142)
- Right bundle branch block (leads V1–V3) (p. 145)
- Subarachnoid haemorrhage
- Pacemaker rhythm (ventricular) (p. 67)

U WAVES

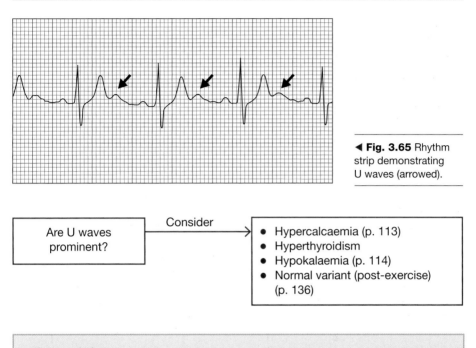

◄ **Fig. 3.65** Rhythm
strip demonstrating
U waves (arrowed).

| Are U waves prominent? | Consider → | • Hypercalcaemia (p. 113)
• Hyperthyroidism
• Hypokalaemia (p. 114)
• Normal variant (post-exercise) (p. 136) |

Hints and tips
• Be wary, prominent U waves may be mistaken for early P waves.

AXIS DEVIATION

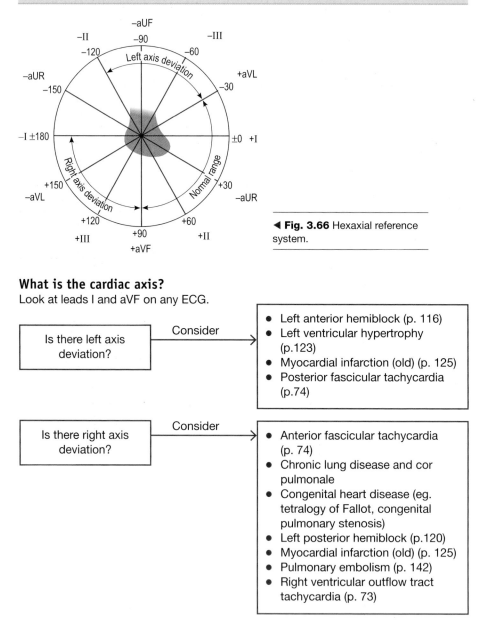

◀ **Fig. 3.66** Hexaxial reference system.

What is the cardiac axis?

Look at leads I and aVF on any ECG.

Is there left axis deviation? — Consider →
- Left anterior hemiblock (p. 116)
- Left ventricular hypertrophy (p.123)
- Myocardial infarction (old) (p. 125)
- Posterior fascicular tachycardia (p.74)

Is there right axis deviation? — Consider →
- Anterior fascicular tachycardia (p. 74)
- Chronic lung disease and cor pulmonale
- Congenital heart disease (eg. tetralogy of Fallot, congenital pulmonary stenosis)
- Left posterior hemiblock (p.120)
- Myocardial infarction (old) (p. 125)
- Pulmonary embolism (p. 142)
- Right ventricular outflow tract tachycardia (p. 73)

An indeterminate axis (sometimes called a North–West axis) is said to occur when the cardiac vector falls between –90° and +180°. This term is also used (particularly by automated reports produced by ECG machines) when all six limb leads appear biphasic and the exact axis cannot be determined.

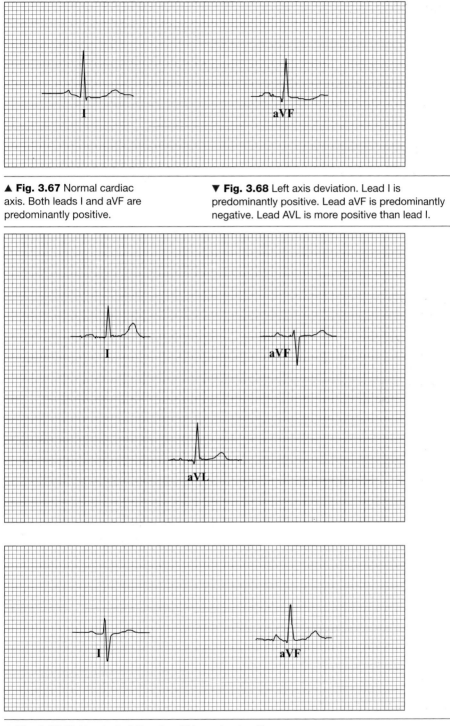

▲ **Fig. 3.67** Normal cardiac axis. Both leads I and aVF are predominantly positive.

▼ **Fig. 3.68** Left axis deviation. Lead I is predominantly positive. Lead aVF is predominantly negative. Lead AVL is more positive than lead I.

▲ **Fig. 3.69** Right axis deviation. Lead I is predominantly negative. Lead aVF is predominantly positive.

3.3
Intervals and waveforms: A–Z of abnormalities

ABERRANT CONDUCTION

See Heart rate and rhythms section, p. 80.

ANEURYSM (LEFT VENTRICULAR)

The presence of persistent ST segment elevation of greater than 1 mm in the precordial leads several days or weeks following an acute myocardial infarction is suggestive of a ventricular aneurysm. This finding is most often associated with an acute anterior myocardial infarction when the ST segment elevation either reappears or persists beyond the subacute phase of MI. Elevation persisting for greater than one week (but more often greater than three months) post MI warrants further investigation because the aneurysmal ventricular wall can be a potential site of left ventricular thrombus and the initiation of ventricular arrhythmias. The test of choice if an aneurysm is suspected is an echocardiogram.

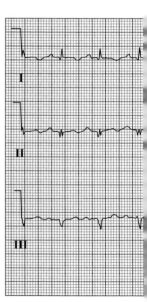

▶ **Fig. 3.70** Left ventricular aneurysm. This ECG was taken from a 62-year-old gentleman during a visit to cardiology outpatients. He had sustained a large anterior MI six weeks before, and was now complaining of persistent chest pain and shortness of breath on moderate exertion.

Key features
- Persistent ST elevation in precordial leads following an acute MI

ASYSTOLE

See Cardiac arrest rhythms (pp. 83–84).

AXIS DEVIATION

See above (p. 104).

BIATRIAL ENLARGEMENT

As the term implies, biatrial enlargement is simply a combination of left and right atrial enlargement (see separate entries for each) and is commonly seen in advanced cardiomyopathy, multivalvular heart disease and in congenital heart disease. P waves are typically both broad and tall, often more than 3 mm tall in limb leads.

BIFASCICULAR BLOCK

When the right bundle branch becomes blocked in combination with a block in either fascicle of the left bundle branch the term bifascicular block is used. Bifascicular block manifests itself on the ECG as right bundle branch block (RBBB) with either left or right axis deviation. If the anterior fascicle is blocked (which is most commonly the case) then left axis deviation will be present. If the posterior fascicle is blocked (rarely) then right axis deviation is seen. (See also Right bundle branch block (p. 145) and section on Cardiac axis (p. 104)).

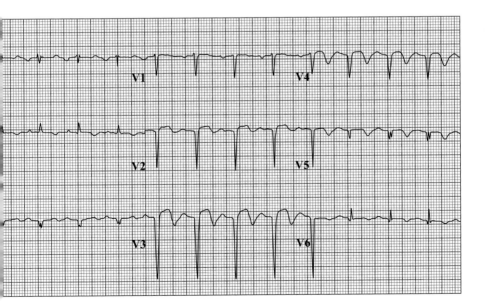

▶ **Fig. 3.71** Bifascicular block: right bundle branch block with left axis deviation. This ECG was recorded in the A&E department from a 60-year-old male who was later admitted due to loss of consciousness. On further questioning, he claimed to have sustained two further episodes of drop attacks over the last 12 months. He smoked 20 cigarettes a day for several years, and was on beta-blocker treatment for hypertension.

Key features
- RBBB with either a left or right axis deviation

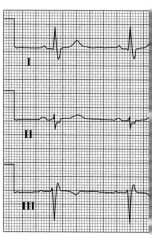

CAUSES
- As for other fascicular blocks.

BRUGADA SYNDROME

See Sudden cardiac death syndromes (p. 147).

BUNDLE BRANCH BLOCK

The presence of block (either complete or incomplete) in the left or right bundle branch causes an abnormal spread of depolarisation through the ventricles and a greater amount of time is taken than usual for ventricular activation to occur. See Left bundle branch block and Right bundle branch block under separate entries (pp. 145 and 119 respectively).

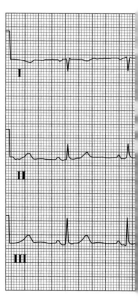

▶ **Fig. 3.72** Dextrocardia (standard leads).

Key features
- Reversed R wave progression
- Inverted complexes in lead I
- Right axis deviation

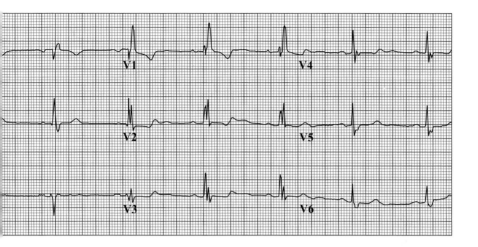

Hints and tips
- Having established that a broad complex QRS is present the key to determining which type of bundle branch block is in evidence – at a glance – is to look for the M-shaped notching (sometimes called "bunny ears") in the chest leads. If there is M-shaped notching of the left-sided chest leads (leads V5 and 6) then LBBB is present. Conversely, M-shaped notching in the right-sided chest leads (V1–V3) indicates RBBB.

DEXTROCARDIA

Dextrocardia is a congenital abnormality in which the heart lies off to the right side of the chest instead of the left. The pattern in both the chest leads and the limb leads are

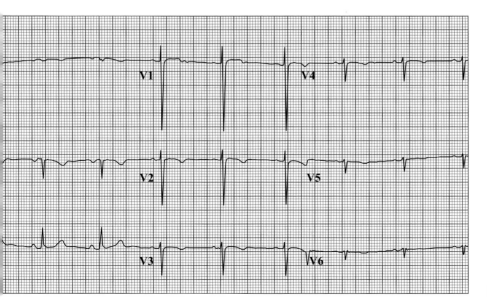

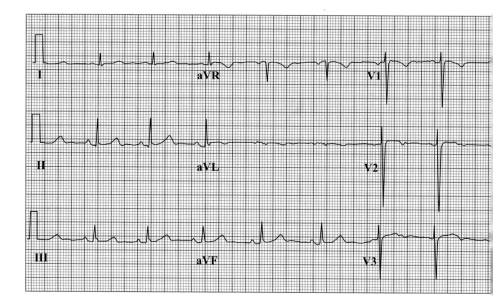

affected. Because of the change in orientation the chest leads show reversed R wave progression with the QRS complexes becoming increasingly negative from V1 through to V6. The limb leads will show an inverted complex in lead I and right axis deviation. In patients with dextrocardia right-sided chest leads (V1R–V6R) should be recorded. (See also Special considerations, p. 32, in Chapter 2.)

Dextrocardia may occur in isolation or in the presence of situs inversus where the abdominal organs are also transposed. Isolated dextrocardia is often associated with other congenital lesions such as transposition of the great vessels, pulmonary stenosis, tetralogy of Fallot, truncus ateriosus and ventricular or atrial septal defects.

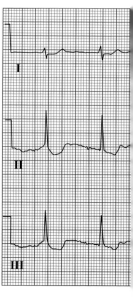

▶ **Fig. 3.74** Atrial fibrillation with digoxin effect demonstrated by downsloping ST segments in leads II, III, aVF and V5 and V6. The ECG was recorded from a 40-year-old man who had been admitted with AF with an initial ventricular rate of 140 bpm. He had been feeling light-headed, and was started on IV, followed by oral digoxin. You should note that these ECG changes are *not* related to ischaemia.

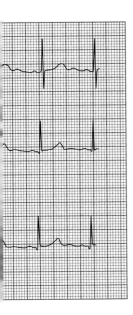

◀ **Fig. 3.73** Dextrocardia with right-sided chest positions results in normal precordial R wave progression and upright complexes in lead I.

DRUG EFFECTS

Changes in the appearance of the ECG and the incidence of particular arrhythmias can be caused by the actions of certain drugs. Unfortunately there are a number of antiarrhythmic drugs which have, as a side-effect, the ability to cause arrhythmias. These are suitably described as pro-arrhythmics.

All of the agents listed in the Vaughan-Williams classification of antiarrhythmic drugs in Table 3.7 below can potentially cause abnormalities on the ECG.

Beta-adrenergic receptor antagonists and some calcium channel blockers may produce sinus bradycardia and varying degrees of AV block.

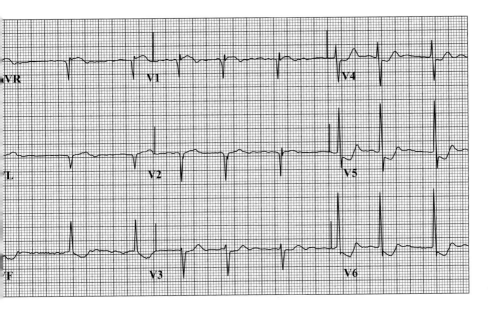

Table 3.7 Vaughan-Williams classification

Class I: Fast sodium channel blockers
- Ia: quinidine, procainamide, disopyramide
- Ib: lidocaine, phenytoin, mexilitene, tocainide
- Ic: encainide, flecainide, propafenone

Class II: ß adrenergic receptor antagonists
- (e.g. propranolol)

Class III: potassium channel blockers
- (e.g. sotalol, amiodarone, dofetilide, ibutilide, bretylium)

Class IV: calcium channel blockers
- (e.g. verapamil, diltiazem, nifedipine)

Digoxin and quinidine-like agents (class Ia) can potentially produce ventricular arrhythmias. Digoxin may cause a short QT interval and a prolonged PR interval on the ECG. T wave inversion and downsloping ST segment depression is produced by the so-called "digoxin effect".

Quinidine has the ability to prolong the QT interval, widen the QRS and precipitate AV nodal blocks.

Drugs such as flecainide may cause bundle branch blocks and, occasionally, ventricular tachycardia. Flecainide can also change pacemaker thresholds and cause loss of capture during pacing.

It is helpful, then, to have to hand details of a patient's current medication when interpreting an ECG.

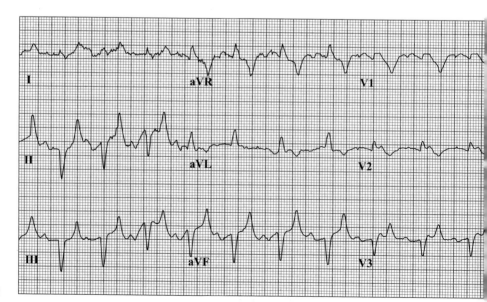

HYPERCALCAEMIA

Definition: Elevated calcium levels in the body.

Table 3.8 Causes and ECG findings in hypercalcaemia

Causes	ECG features
Drugs such as thiazide diuretics	Short QT interval
Excessive vitamin D intake	Prolongation of PR interval and QRS
Hyperparathyroidism	complex (less commonly)
Malignancy	Ventricular arrhythmias
Milk-alkali syndrome	
Sarcoidosis	
Thyrotoxicosis	

HYPERKALAEMIA

Definition: Elevated potassium levels in the body.

Table 3.9 Causes and ECG findings in hyperkalaemia

Causes	ECG features
Renal failure	Tall T waves $\geq$ associated R waves in more than
Acidosis	one lead (potassium levels between 5.5–6.5 mmol/l)
Shock	+/–
Overadministration of potassium	Low amplitude "flattened" P waves
Potassium-sparing diuretics	Prolongation of PR interval (potassium levels
Angiotensin-converting enzyme	between 6.5–7.5 mmol/l)
inhibitors	+/–
	Broad QRS complex (potassium levels between
	7.0–8.0 mmol/l)
	+/–
	Ventricular arrhythmias, asystole (potassium
	levels between 8.0–10.0 mmol/l)

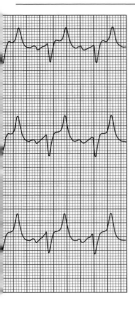

◀ **Fig. 3.75** This is hyperkalaemia secondary to renal failure and potassium-retaining medication as demonstrated by peaked T waves in all leads and widespread broadening of the QRS complexes. The ECG was taken from a 58-year-old male with hypertension, peripheral vascular disease and heart failure. His drug history included ramipril 10 mg od and spironolactone 25 mg od. His serum creatinine was noted to be 350 µmol/L.

113

HYPOCALCAEMIA

Definition: depleted calcium levels in the body.

Table 3.10 Causes and ECG findings in hypocalcaemia

Causes	ECG features
Chronic renal failure	Prolonged QT interval
Vitamin D deficiency	T wave flattening or inversion (less common)
Hypoparathyroidism	Ventricular arrhythmias
Parathyroidectomy	
Pseudohypoparathyroidism	
Respiratory or metabolic alkalosis	
Drugs (e.g.calcitonin, heparin, glucagon)	

HYPOKALAEMIA

Definition: depleted potassium levels in the body.

Table 3.11 Causes and ECG findings in hypokalaemia

Causes	ECG features
Drugs (e.g. diuretics,	Peaked P waves (severe cases)
Insulin, beta$_2$ agonists)	Prolonged PR interval
Vomiting/diarrhoea	Broad, flat T waves
Starvation or malnutrition	ST depression
Renal tubular acidosis	Prolonged QT interval
Conn's syndrome (hyperaldosteronism)	Prominent U waves
Cushing's syndrome (hypercortisolism)	Ventricular and supraventricular arrhythmias

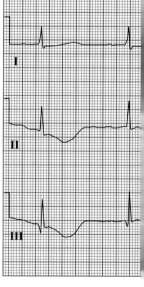

▶ **Fig. 3.76** Hypokalaemia. There are prolonged PR and QT intervals, widespread ST depression and prominent U waves seen in lead V2. The ECG was recorded two days post-admission from a 40-year-old patient who had recently returned from a holiday in South America. He was admitted to hospital with severe diarrhoea and vomiting.

HYPOTHERMIA

The most characteristic feature of hypothermia on an ECG is the development of a J wave producing a notched appearance in the QRS complex. This is best seen in left-sided chest leads and the size of the wave is thought to correlate with the severity of the hypothermia.

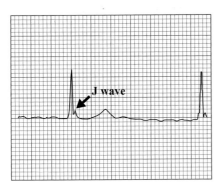

◀ **Fig. 3.77** J wave in hypothermia.

ECG features associated with hypothermia

- Muscle tremor artefact
- Bradycardias (including atrial fibrillation with slow ventricular response)
- Prolongation of PR, QRS and QT intervals
- J waves
- Ventricular arrhythmias
- Asystole.

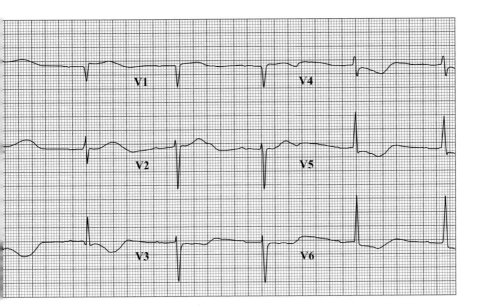

LEFT ANTERIOR HEMIBLOCK

As you will remember from the first chapter the left bundle branch is divided into two portions, namely the anterior and posterior fascicles. A block in either of these fascicles is termed a hemiblock and the result is an axis deviation on the ECG.

In left anterior hemiblock the cardiac axis shifts to the left and is manifested as a left axis deviation (≥ –30°). (Compare left posterior hemiblock below.)

The anterior fascicle is long and thin and has just a single blood supply making it more vulnerable than the posterior fascicle. Hence block in the anterior fascicle is more common.

CAUSES

- Congenital heart disease
- Cardiac surgery
- Fibrosis of conducting system
- Ischaemic heart disease
- Myocardial infarction.

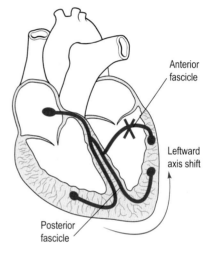

▶ **Fig. 3.78** Axis shift in left anterior hemiblock.

Hints and tips

- Before diagnosing left anterior hemiblock from the ECG you should first be sure no other causes of left axis deviation exist (see separate section on cardiac axis (p. 104)).

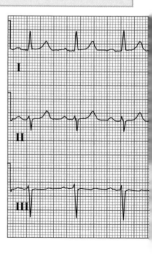

▶ **Fig. 3.79** Left anterior hemiblock.

Key features

- Left axis deviation
- Deep terminal S waves in leads II and III
- QRS may be slightly prolonged (up to 0.11 secs)

LEFT ATRIAL ENLARGEMENT

Otherwise known as P mitrale because it is often associated with mitral valve disease, an enlarged left atrium produces P waves in excess of two small squares (or 0.08secs) wide and which may be bifid (or notched) in appearance. The P waves are wider than normal because the spread of depolarisation takes longer due to the larger chamber size.

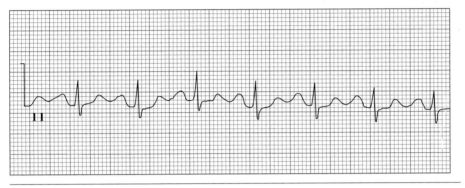

▲ **Fig. 3.80** Left atrial enlargement. This ECG was taken from a patient with known mitral valve prolapse who had been complaining of increasing shortness of breath during an outpatient visit. She had a loud pan-systolic murmur audible in the apex. An echocardiogram showed moderate–severe mitral regurgitation.

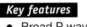

Key features
- Broad P wave, duration > 0.08 secs

CAUSES

- Atrial fibrillation
- Aortic valve disease
- Cardiomyopathy
- Hypertension
- Mitral valve disease.

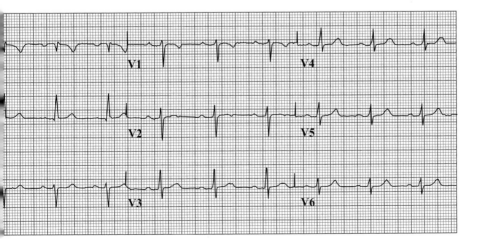

Enlargement of the left atrium does not require any treatment on its own – treatment is directed towards the underlying cause.

> ### Hints and tips
> - P waves are best seen in leads II and V1. In lead V1 left atrial enlargement tends to produce a biphasic P wave with both a positive and negative component
> - In atrial fibrillation left atrial enlargement may still be discerned despite the absence of P waves if there are coarse fibrillation waves (>1 mm) present in leads V1 or V2.

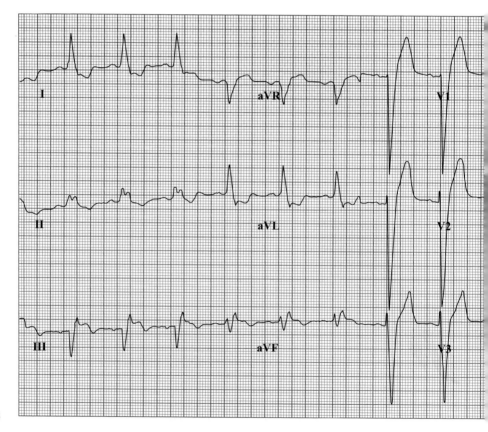

LEFT BUNDLE BRANCH BLOCK

Left bundle branch block is described as either complete or incomplete. In complete left bundle branch block the ventricular septum depolarises from right to left which accounts for the loss of septal Q waves in leads V4–6. Activation of the ventricles via the right bundle branch causes a broader than normal QRS complex in all leads with the characteristic M-shape notching seen in the lateral leads.

When conduction through the left bundle branch is delayed (but not blocked) a pattern of incomplete LBBB is seen. The QRS duration is in excess of 0.10 secs (2.5 small squares) but less than 0.12 secs (3 small squares). This may be difficult to appreciate in terms of time – especially when you are counting *between* small squares – but the ECG pattern is quite distinctive.

New onset LBBB can be a presenting feature of acute myocardial infarction and the patient should be treated accordingly. The causes of pre-existing LBBB are listed below.

CAUSES

- Cardiomyopathy
- Hypertension
- Ischaemic heart disease
- Left ventricular hypertrophy
- Myocarditis.

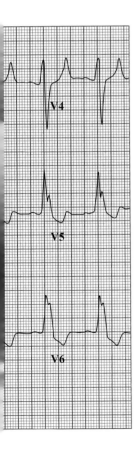

◀ **Fig. 3.81** Left bundle branch block. This patient was a 48-year-old man referred for a specialist opinion on the basis of this ECG, taken during a routine health check. His blood pressure was 120/75. The young man reported only mild shortness of breath on exertion. A subsequent echocardiogram revealed findings consistent with dilated cardiomyopathy.

Key features

- QRS duration > 0.12 secs (or 3 small squares) in all leads
- Characteristic M-shaped notching seen in leads V5 and V6

119

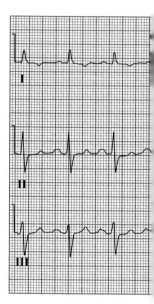

▶ **Fig. 3.82** Left bundle branch block (incomplete).

Key features
- QRS duration of between 0.10 – 0.12 secs

LEFT POSTERIOR HEMIBLOCK

The posterior fascicle of the left bundle branch is anatomically short and thick with a double blood supply making it less susceptible to block than the anterior fascicle. In left posterior hemiblock the cardiac axis shifts to the right and is manifested as a right axis deviation (> 90°) on the ECG.

CAUSES
- Cardiomyopathy
- Ischaemic heart disease.

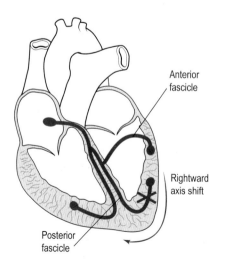

Anterior fascicle

Rightward axis shift

Posterior fascicle

◀ **Fig. 3.83** Axis shift in left posterior hemiblock.

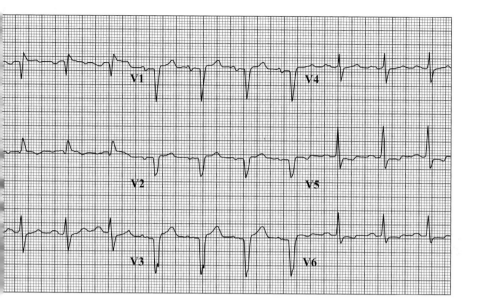

LEFT VENTRICULAR HYPERTROPHY (LVH)

Due to the increased left ventricular muscle mass, greater positive R wave voltages are seen in the left-sided chest leads (V5 and 6) and greater negative S wave voltages may also be seen in the right-sided chest leads (V1 or V2). LVH is suggested if the sum of the S wave in V1 and the R wave in V5 or 6 ≥ 35 mm.

Typically there is an associated characteristic "strain" pattern present which manifests itself as downsloping ST depression. This is not associated with ischaemia and is more to do with the abnormal repolarisation of the hypertrophied left ventricle. In about 50% of patients left axis deviation may also be present.

CAUSES

- Aortic stenosis
- Athletic heart
- Coarctation of aorta
- Fabry's disease
- Hypertension
- Hypertrophic obstructive cardiomyopathy.

Hints and tips

- Before diagnosing left posterior hemiblock from the ECG you should first be sure no other causes of right axis deviation exist (see separate section on cardiac axis (p. 104)).

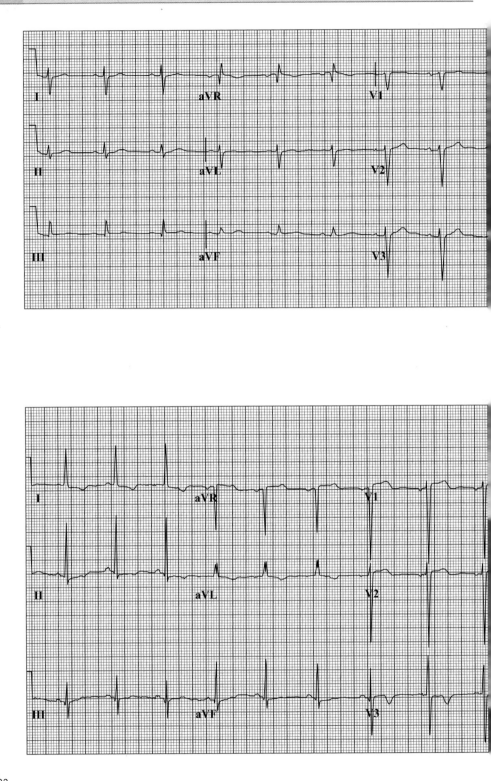

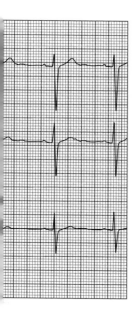

◀ **Fig. 3.84** Left posterior hemiblock.

Key features

- Right axis deviation
- QRS may be slightly prolonged (up to 0.11 secs)

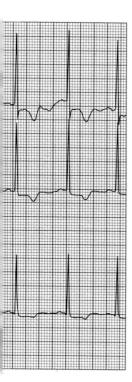

◀ **Fig. 3.85** This ECG shows deep anterior S waves and tall lateral R waves with ST and T wave changes. The ECG was recorded from a 57-year-old man with longstanding poorly controlled hypertension who had been referred to the nephrology outpatients for investigation of a raised creatinine. He had protein ++ on dipstick urinalysis. The ECG represents LVH with a history suggestive of target organ damage.

Key features

- Total of S wave in V1 + R wave in V5/6 ≥ 35 mm
- Presence of strain pattern
- Possible left axis deviation

LONG QT SYNDROME

See Sudden cardiac death syndromes (p. 147).

LOWN–GANONG–LEVINE SYNDROME

This syndrome is characterised by the presence of an accessory pathway (named the bundle of James) through which conduction from the atria to the ventricles bypasses the AV node. It appears on the surface ECG simply as a short PR interval. Patients with Lown–Ganong–Levine syndrome present the same risks for paroxysmal tachycardias as patients with Wolf–Parkinson–White syndrome.

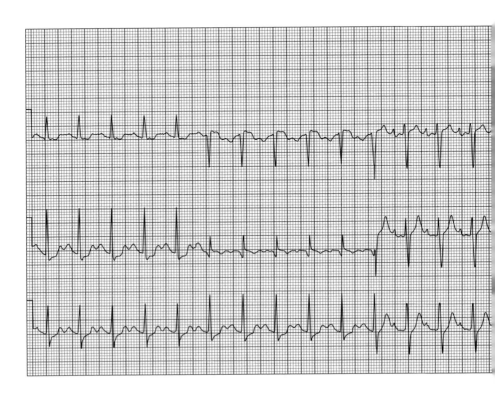

MYOCARDIAL ISCHAEMIA AND INFARCTION

Myocardial ischaemia and infarction are a part of the same disease spectrum, namely the so-called acute coronary syndromes, and are typically divided into non-ST elevation disorders – including unstable angina and non-ST elevation MI (NSTEMI) – and ST elevation myocardial infarction (STEMI). Typically they are differentiated in terms of clinical history, ECG findings and biochemical markers.

Ideally an ECG should be recorded when the patient is symptomatic. The ECG changes associated with the acute coronary syndromes include ST segment depression, T wave inversion, the development of bundle branch block and ST segment elevation. Occasionally, however, the ECG may be entirely normal.

ST segment depression

ST segment depression, particularly on exertion, is strongly suggestive of myocardial ischaemia. Both the magnitude and morphology of the changes in the ST segment help to differentiate normal ST changes on exercise from true ischaemia. Rapidly upsloping ST depression is nearly always normal whereas downsloping or horizontal (planar) depression is strongly indicative of coronary artery disease (see section on The ECG and exercise testing in Chapter 2, p. 35).

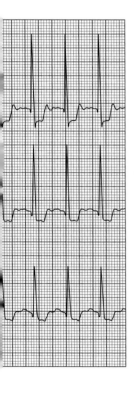

◀ **Fig. 3.86** Note the presence of horizontal ST depression in lead V4 and downsloping ST changes in leads V5 and 6. The ECG was recorded during an exercise test from a 43-year-old male smoker with a 3-month history of vague chest pain during swimming who had presented to the Rapid Access Chest Pain Clinic. The test was stopped at stage 2 of the full Bruce protocol because the patient developed chest pain and felt faint.

T wave changes

Typically T waves may become inverted or flat. When interpreting an ECG for ischaemia it is important to rule out any other possible causes of T wave changes such as normal variants, myocarditis, left ventricular hypertrophy and the effects of drugs such as digoxin all of which cause the T waves to become inverted.

Deep symmetrical inversion of T waves reflects the presence of subendocardial ischaemia and is often a feature of non-ST elevation MI.

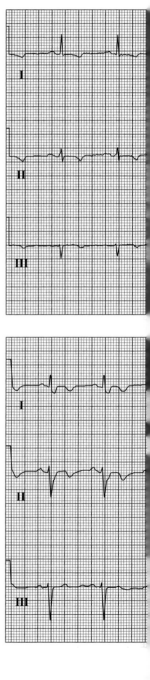

▶ **Fig. 3.87** This ECG shows widespread T wave inversion and was recorded from a 60-year-old lady with a history of increasing shortness of breath on exertion. A treadmill test later demonstrated significant ST depression in the anterolateral leads accompanied with moderate dyspnoea. The lady was later referred for angiography.

▶ **Fig. 3.88** On the fourth day after he was admitted with unstable angina, a 72-year-old male developed severe central chest pain with vomiting. The nurse on the coronary care unit was prompt to take his ECG. Note the deep symmetrical ST and T wave changes in leads V4–V6. Blood taken 12 hours after symptoms revealed raised troponin and CK levels. The patient was diagnosed with non-ST elevation MI.

ST elevation

ST elevation occurring only transiently is a feature typically associated with Prinzmetal's angina. Persistent ST elevation characterises an evolving myocardial infarction.

ST elevation myocardial infarction (STEMI)

Severe, acute, ischaemia is caused by occlusion of a coronary vessel (usually by a thrombus or the rupture of an atherosclerotic plaque). During coronary artery occlusion

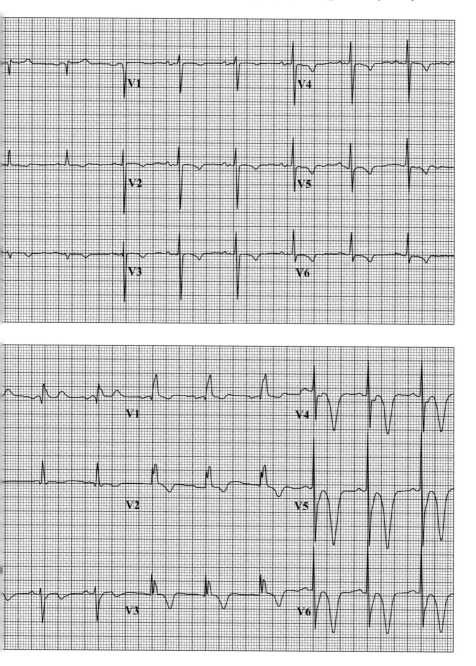

a current of injury appears on the surface ECG manifested as acute elevation of the ST segment. If not quickly corrected with thrombolysis or emergency PCI (percutaneous coronary intervention) myocardial necrosis results.

Localisation of the site of infarction

Unlike ST depression in ischaemia, ST elevation on the ECG *does* relate to the underlying cardiac anatomy. The associated myocardial territories and the coronary artery involved in the myocardial injury correlate well with the ECG leads which "look at" that particular region of the heart (Table 3.12).

The most commonly affected areas are the anterior and inferior regions. Anteroseptal ST elevation strongly indicates disease of the left anterior descending artery. Isolated inferior ST elevation indicates right coronary or distal circumflex artery occlusions. A lateral infarct pattern is associated predominantly with disease to the proximal circumflex.

ST elevation should occur in two or more anatomically contiguous leads (i.e. two leads that look at the same surface of the heart).

It is important to be able to differentiate the different causes of ST segment elevation on an ECG because the clinical approach will be different. Other causes of ST elevation on an ECG are:

- Brugada syndrome
- Early repolarisation
- Left bundle branch block
- Left ventricular aneurysm
- Pericarditis
- Variant (Printzmetal's) angina.

Left bundle branch block and acute MI

LBBB typically renders the ECG uninterpretable for ischaemia. However the following are thought to be specific indicators of acute ischaemic changes in LBBB.

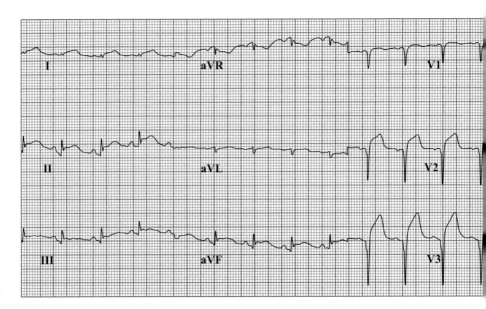

Table 3.12 Localisation of site of infarction

ECG leads demonstrating ST elevation	Anatomical location
V1–V4	Anterior
V2–V4	Anteroseptal
V2–V6	Anterolateral
II, III, aVF	Inferior
II, III, aVF, V5, V6	Inferolateral
V7, V8, V9 (ST depression V1–V3)	Posterior
II, III, aVF, V1 + right-sided chest leads	Right ventricle

- *Inappropriate concordance* – the presence of ST segment elevation in ECG leads with predominantly positive QRS complexes (in LBBB these are largely the inferolateral leads) or ST segment depression in leads with predominantly negative QRS complexes (in LBBB these are the anterior leads).
- *Extreme ST segment elevation* – greater than 5 mm in anterior leads.

Reciprocal ST depression

Reciprocal ST depression is a feature of acute MI and is demonstrated in leads away from the site of infarction. It is thought to be due to "mirror-image" changes so that positive potentials recorded in leads facing the site of injury are "mirrored" by negative changes in the leads opposite. For instance it is not uncommon to observe ST depression in leads II, III and aVF (inferior leads) during an acute anterior MI affecting leads V1–V4. The precise mechanism for these reciprocal changes is poorly understood but their presence on the ECG should aid interpretation.

Resolution of acute changes

ST elevation begins to diminish either as soon as the intervention has taken effect or as the infarct progresses and Q waves begin to develop. ST elevation in inferior MI may

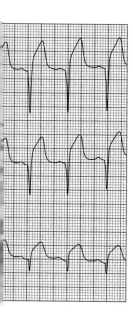

◀ **Fig. 3.89** Extensive resolving myocardial infarction. Note the presence of widespread ST elevation accompanied by pathological Q waves in leads V2 to V6.

take as long as two weeks to fully resolve. ST changes associated with anterior MI may take even longer and even persist indefinitely in the presence of a left ventricular aneurysm.

Q waves may start to develop as soon as two hours after the onset of the ST changes but more usually take between 12–24 hours. The presence of pathological Q waves, often along with T wave inversion, remain permanently on the patient's ECG once the

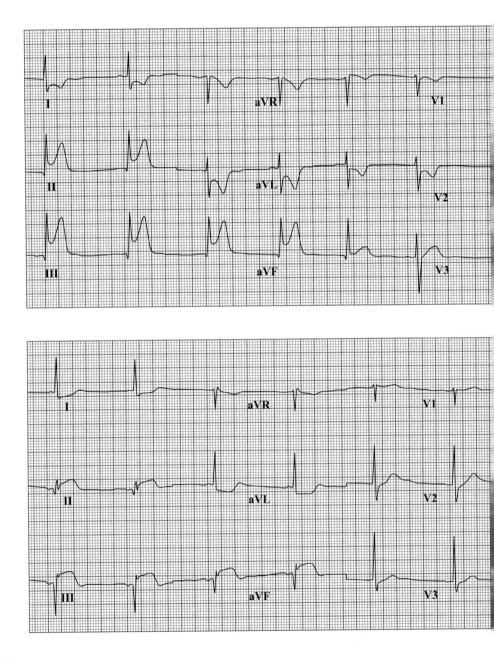

infarct is complete. The Q wave is thought to form because infarcted tissue is effectively electrically inert. This dead tissue acts like a "window" through which the ECG records electrical activity from other areas of the heart. Depolarisation is therefore directed away from the recording electrode and hence appears inverted on the ECG. This inversion forms the Q wave.

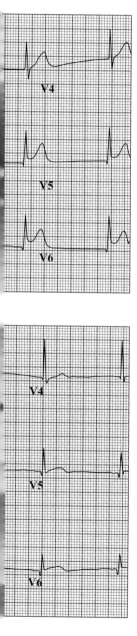

◄ **Fig. 3.90** Acute inferolateral myocardial infarction with reciprocal ST depression in leads I, aVL and V2.

◄ **Fig. 3.91** This is the same patient 24 hours later. Note that the ST elevation is now resolving and Q waves have developed in leads III and aVF.

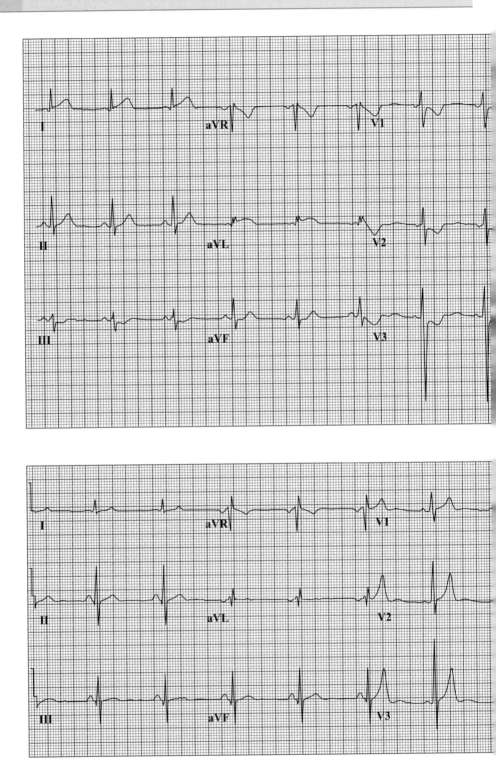

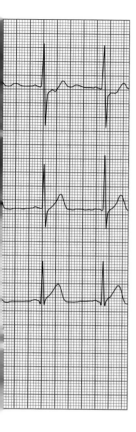

◀ **Fig. 3.92** Acute posterolateral myocardial infarction evidenced by the presence of downsloping ST depression and tall R waves in leads V1 to V3 and ST elevation in leads I and aVL.

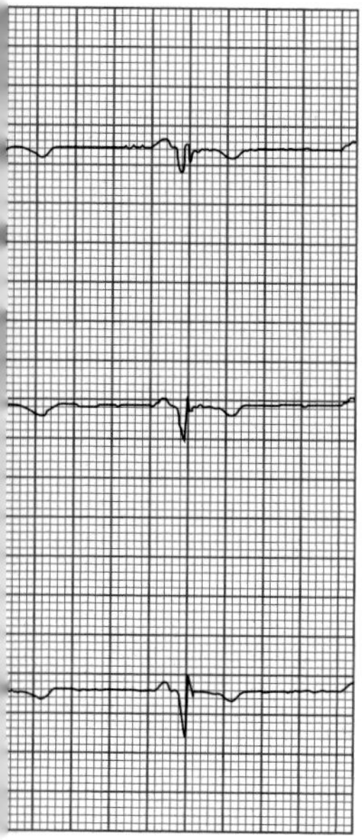

◀ **Fig. 3.93** This ECG was taken from the same patient 5 days later when he attended for his pre-discharge exercise test. Note that the technician has recorded leads V7–V9 which reveal posterior Q waves and almost fully resolved ST segment changes.

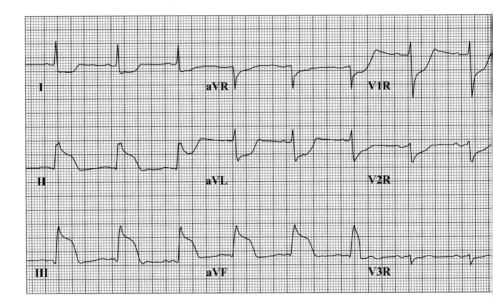

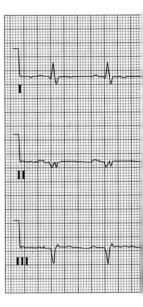

▶ **Fig. 3.95** Old inferoposterior MI as demonstrated by Q waves in leads II, III and aVF and the tall R wave in lead V1.

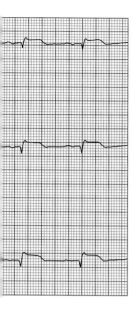

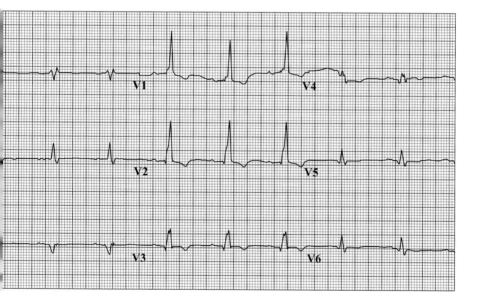

◄ **Fig. 3.94** This recording includes right-sided chest leads and shows an acute inferior myocardial infarction with right ventricular involvement.

NORMAL VARIANTS

If you set yourself the task of collecting as many "normal" ECGs as possible it would soon become apparent just how difficult it is to find two normal ECGs which look the same because there are so many different forms of normal variations out there.

Normal variants are frequently observed in healthy individuals and it is useful to be able to recognise them so that no confusion arises from their discovery.

The tracing below is a typical example of what a "normal" 12 lead ECG looks like. Memorise this ECG and compare it with every other ECG you ever see!

Normal variations in the PR interval

A short PR interval may be normal in healthy children and young adults. Rarely first degree AV block or nocturnal Mobitz type I (Wenckebach) AV block is also observed in this age group.

Normal variations in the QRS complex

Low voltage QRS complexes are often measured from obese patients due to the greater amount of body tissue across the chest.

High left ventricular QRS voltages are often seen in the left-sided chest leads in young adults and in very slim patients.

Normal variations in the ST segment

Early repolarisation (sometimes called high take-off) is a normal finding in young healthy individuals and in healthy black males. In this instance there is elevation of the ST seg-

NON-SPECIFIC INTRAVENTRICULAR CONDUCTION DELAY

This is a non-specific widening of the QRS complex which does not fit any bundle branch block pattern which occurs secondary to conditions such as left ventricular hypertrophy and cardiomyopathy.

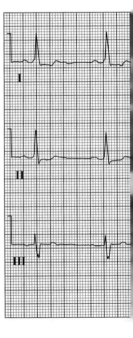

▶ **Fig. 3.96** Non-specific IVC.

Key features

- QRS greater than 0.12 seconds
- Does not fit any bundle branch block pattern

ment at the J-point which can occur in any lead but particularly in the anterolateral chest leads (V2–V6).

Normal variations in the T wave

T wave inversion in leads V4–V6 is a common finding in athletic individuals and in some young people and is termed "athletic T wave change". Deformed or inverted T waves in leads V1–V3 is also a common finding in children which may persist into adulthood. In this case the term "persistent juvenile T wave pattern" is used.

Miscellaneous variations

You may have noticed that many of the normal variants are related to young healthy people who perhaps shouldn't be having an ECG in the first place! Additionally, children and young adults may also demonstrate right axis deviation, a short QT interval, sinus arrhythmia and (occasionally) a wandering atrial pacemaker.

Sinus bradycardia is a normal response in a heart conditioned by exercise and is thus a common finding in athletic individuals.

One last normal variation is the finding of a significant-looking Q wave and/or T wave inversion in lead III. The R wave may also appear biphasic. This is a respiratory variation termed "lead III$_R$". If you run a rhythm strip and get the patient to take a big breath in, you will see that the R wave "pops up", the Q wave disappears and the T wave becomes upright.

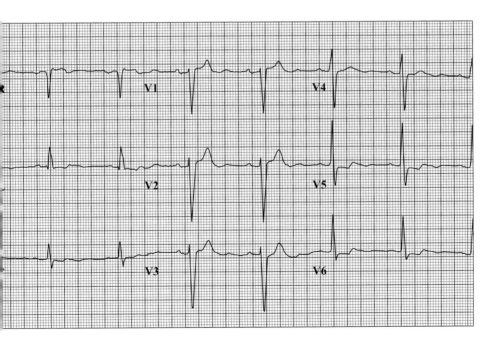

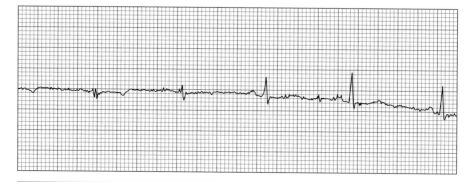

▲ **Fig. 3.97** This rhythm strip was recorded in lead III and shows the presence of a poorly defined QRS complex with T wave inversion. The patient was asked to take a big breath in and hold and the third beat shows the transition to a more prominent R wave and T wave normalisation.

▶ **Fig.3.98** Normal 12 lead ECG.

Key features

- Heart rate between 60–100 bpm
- One P wave for every QRS complex (sinus rhythm)
- Normal P wave height and duration (2.5 mm and 0.08 secs)
- Normal PR interval (between 0.12–0.20 secs)
- Normal QRS duration and height in precordial leads (≤ 0.10 secs and ≤ 25 mm)
- Normal R wave progression (chest leads)
- Normal QRS axis (between +90° and −30° in limb leads)
- Isoelectric ST segments
- T waves pointing same direction as associated R wave

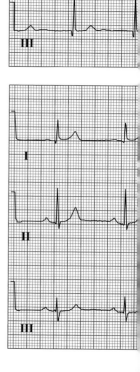

▶ **Fig.3.99** Early repolarisation throughout the chest leads. This is differentiated from ST elevation by the presence of S waves in the leads V3 and V4.

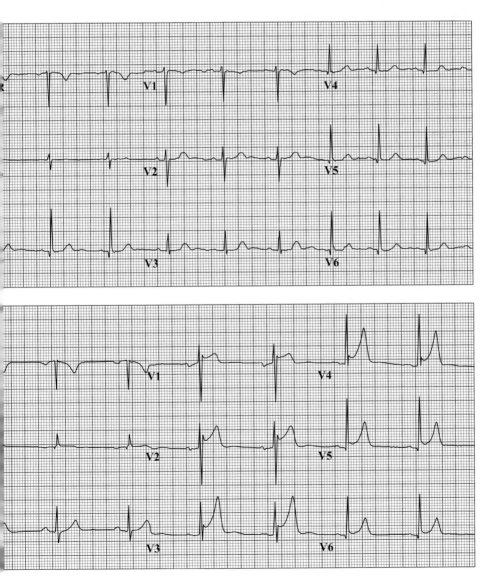

THE PAEDIATRIC ECG

A discussion of the many complexities of paediatric ECG analysis is beyond the scope of this book. The following, however, is intended to be a brief mention of a few of the things you should bear in mind.

Resting heart rates in the neonate are usually around 140 bpm. By the age of one year the resting heart rate falls to around 120 bpm and to 100 bpm by the age of five. Adult values are usually reached by the age of 10. It is not unusual to see sinus tachycardia in active babies and infants up to 240 bpm. Sinus arrhythmia, often marked, is very common. Second degree AV block (Wenckebach phenomenon) is occasionally seen in otherwise healthy children.

Normal features of paediatric ECGs
- Heart rate > 100 bpm
- Short P wave duration and PR interval
- Inferior and lateral Q waves
- Short QRS duration, dominant right precordial R waves, QRS axis > +90°
- Short QT interval
- T wave inversion leads V1–V3.

Analysis of the paediatric ECG is similar, *in general*, to that of the adult ECG *bearing in mind* the age-related differences listed above. Note that genuine abnormalities are unusual particularly in children without a history of congenital defects. Expert advice should always be sought if you suspect an abnormality is present.

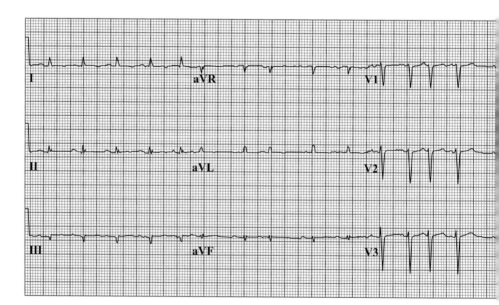

PERICARDIAL EFFUSION

Excessive build-up of fluid in the sac around the heart produces two distinct ECG findings. Firstly, because of the extra fluid, and therefore greater distance between the electrode and the heart, low voltage QRS complexes are common. Secondly a phenomenon known as ventricular electrical alternans is sometimes seen. Because of the expansion of the pericardium due to the extra fluid the heart is allowed more movement towards and away from the electrodes as it beats. This produces QRS complexes of alternating amplitude on the ECG.

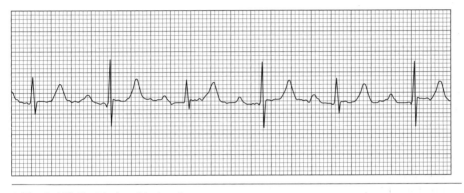

▲ **Fig. 3.100** Electrical ventricular alternans.

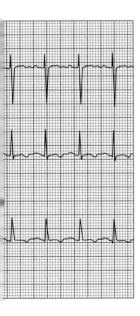

◀ **Fig. 3.101** This ECG was obtained from a patient with end-stage renal failure who was being treated with CAPD. His wife had brought him to casualty after he had woken up with severe pallor, shortness of breath and dizziness. Note the presence of sinus tachycardia with small QRS complexes throughout. The patient was diagnosed with pericardial effusion secondary to chronic renal failure with pericardial tamponade.

Key features

- Low voltage QRS complexes
- Ventricular electrical alternans (occasionally)
- Sinus tachycardia

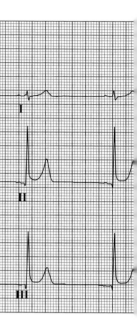

▶ **Fig. 3.102** Pericarditis. This ECG was taken from a 39-year-old hypertensive male with a strong family history of coronary artery disease who had been admitted urgently to hospital with severe chest pain. He was given aspirin and sublingual nitrate spray with no relief of his symptoms. The SHO asked his registrar to review the case; on seeing the ECG, the registrar immediately stopped all treatment and suggested a diagnosis of pericarditis. The ECG shows widespread "saddle-shaped" ST elevation which is more marked in leads II, III and aVF.

Key features

- Widespread ST elevation
- Characteristic saddle shaped ST segments
- Absence of reciprocal ST depression

PERICARDITIS

Patients presenting with pericarditis describe retrosternal chest pain and demonstrate ST segment elevation on their ECG. It is therefore important to be able to distinguish pericarditis from acute myocardial infarction both clinically and electrocardiographically.

Electrocardiographically the ST segment elevation is widespread involving many, if not all, lead groups (with the exception of lead aVR where the ST segment may appear depressed). The ST elevation is characteristically "saddle-shaped", that is, concave upwards in appearance and there will be no reciprocal ST segment depression. PR segment depression may also be seen and, occasionally, a sinus tachycardia is evident. The presence of a large pericardial effusion may additionally produce findings similar to those already described above.

In the later stages the ST elevation returns to baseline and T wave inversion occurs which may persist for weeks or months. Note that Q waves do not develop.

PULMONARY EMBOLISM

ECG changes during an acute pulmonary embolism tend to occur within the first 24–48 hours and are transient in nature. Hence the timing and frequency of ECG recording is important. Patients presenting with a small pulmonary embolus are likely to have a normal trace. Findings associated with a large pulmonary embolism include:

- Sinus tachycardia
- S wave in lead I with a Q wave and T wave inversion in lead III (the frequently quoted S1 Q3 T3 pattern)
- Right atrial enlargement
- Right axis deviation

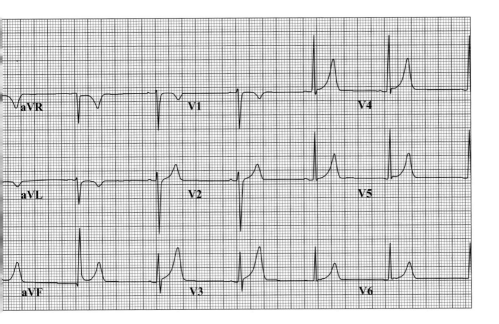

- T wave inversion in leads V1–V3
- Incomplete or complete right bundle branch block (less commonly)
- Atrial arrhythmias.

Note that the S1 Q3 T3 pattern is only seen in around 12% of patients presenting with a massive pulmonary embolus.

RIGHT ATRIAL ENLARGEMENT

Tall, peaked P waves (> 2.5 mm) in leads II, III and aVF are suggestive of right atrial enlargement. It is sometimes called P pulmonale because it is often associated with

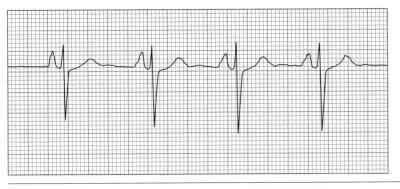

▲ **Fig. 3.103** Right atrial enlargement.

Key features

- Tall, peaked P waves (> 2.5 mm) in inferior leads

> **Hints and tips**
> - Severe hypokalaemia may also cause tall peaked P waves and should be excluded.

various pulmonary diseases. When enlargement of the right atrium is due to congenital heart disease, the term used is P congenitale.

CAUSES

- Atrial fibrillation
- Atrial septal defect
- Cardiomyopathies
- Chronic right heart failure of any cause.

- Pulmonary hypertension – primary, or secondary to chronic lung disease or chronic left-to-right shunt
- Tricuspid valve stenosis and regurgitation

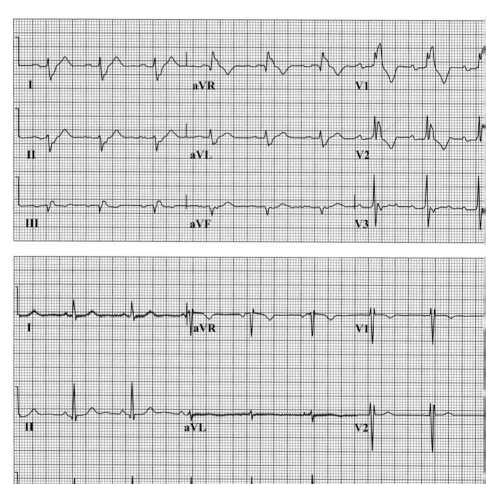

RIGHT BUNDLE BRANCH BLOCK (RBBB)

In RBBB the ventricular septum depolarises in the normal way but activation of the right ventricle is delayed. This produces a characteristic rSR' (or M-shaped notching) in right precordial leads (V1–V3) and deep slurred S waves in the lateral leads.

When conduction through the right bundle branch is delayed (but not blocked) a pattern of incomplete RBBB is seen.

CAUSES

- Atrial septal defects
- Brugada syndrome
- Ebstein's anomaly
- Pulmonary embolism
- Radiotherapy of the chest wall
- Surgical interventions to the right ventricle.

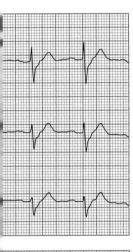

◀ **Fig. 3.104** Complete right bundle branch block with right axis deviation and first degree heart block. This ECG is also an example of trifascicular block.

Key features

- QRS duration > 0.12 secs
- M-shaped notching in leads V1–V3

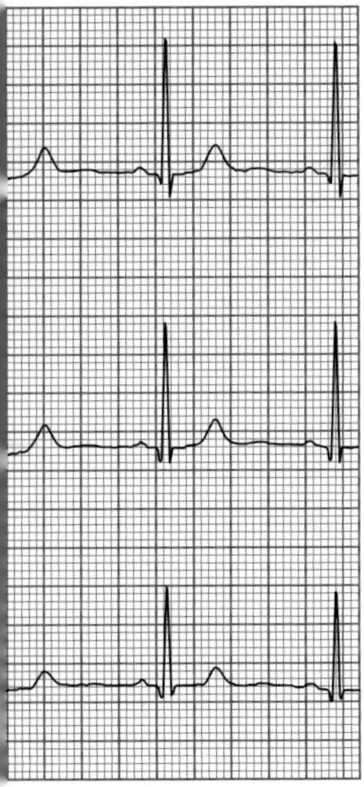

◀ **Fig. 3.105** Right bundle branch block (incomplete).

Key features

- QRS duration of between 0.10–0.12 secs.
- rSR' present in leads V1–V3

145

RIGHT VENTRICULAR HYPERTROPHY (RVH)

The ECG is relatively insensitive to cases of mild RVH and in such circumstances may appear normal. However, in the presence of significant hypertrophy the cardiac axis undergoes a rightward shift with a dominant R wave appearing in lead V1. Occasionally a strain pattern emerges manifested as downsloping T wave inversion in the anterior (right-sided) chest leads.

CAUSES

- Pulmonary hypertension
  - Primary
  - Secondary – chronic lung disease (e.g. interstitial lung disease, pulmonary fibrosis), mitral valve disease, left heart failure, congenital left-to-right shunts (e.g. atrial or ventricular septal defects), in connective tissue disease (e.g. systemic sclerosis), HIV infection, appetite-suppressing drugs

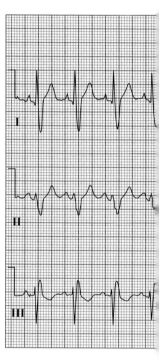

▶ **Fig. 3.106** Right ventricular hypertrophy. A 35-year-old male manual labourer was referred by his GP to the cardiology outpatient clinic because of worsening shortness of breath on exertion. He had surgery about a year previously for "a hole in the heart" which he had since birth and this was his ECG.

Key features
- Right axis deviation ($\geq +110°$)
- Dominant R wave V1

- Congenital right ventricular outflow tract obstruction e.g. Fallot's tetrology, pulmonary valve stenosis
- Transposition of great arteries, where right ventricle is connected to systemic circulation.

SUDDEN CARDIAC DEATH SYNDROMES

Brugada syndrome

Brugada syndrome is a sudden death syndrome caused by an autosomal dominant gene which brings about changes in sodium ion transport mechanisms in the right ventricle. Mutations in the SCN5A gene of the sodium channel cause the channel to malfunction. The condition is consequently made worse by the use of sodium-channel blocking agents. It is associated with a right bundle branch block pattern ECG with ST elevation in the right-sided chest leads (which may be only transient), sudden cardiac death (most commonly secondary to ventricular fibrillation) and the absence of struc-

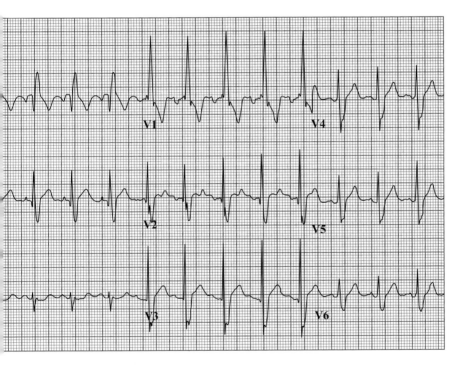

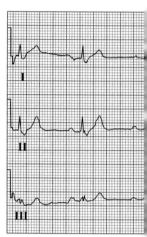

▶ **Fig. 3.107** Brugada syndrome. This ECG was taken from a young man who was diagnosed with asthma at an appointment with a lung physician. However his ECG was so unusual he was sent for an echocardiogram, which was entirely normal. The young man gave a history of sudden death in young family members and was subsequently referred to a cardiologist.

Key features

- Right bundle branch block pattern
- Anterior lead ST elevation

tural heart disease. Brugada syndrome may develop at any age but typically develops in middle life.

Presently, antiarrhythmic therapy has not proved successful and the only potential treatment is the implantation of an implantable defibrillator.

Long QT syndrome

This disorder may be either acquired or genetic and consists of a clinical combination of a long QT interval (greater than 0.43 seconds), episodes of syncope, ventricular tachycardia, torsades de pointes and sudden cardiac death.

The acquired form of long QT syndrome may be caused by:

- Drugs (antiarrhythmic types I or III, antipsychotics, some antibiotics and some non-sedating antihistamines)
- Neurological problems
- Cardiac ischaemia
- Metabolic disorders.

There are two genetic types of long QT syndrome, the Romano–Ward syndrome and the Jervell and Lange–Nielson syndrome, and these are rare.

Romano–Ward syndrome is an autosomal dominant disease whereas Jervell and Lange-Neilsen syndrome is an autosomal recessive characteristic that is also responsible for high-tone deafness. In both syndromes patients are largely young and present with syncopal attacks particularly related to exertion or stress.

Beta blockade is useful for reducing syncopal episodes in these patients. Alternative therapies include the insertion of an implantable defibrillator or cervical sympathectomy.

Arrhythmogenic right ventricular dysplasia (ARVD)

This is thought to be an autosomal dominant condition (although the precise genetic mechanisms are not yet fully understood) characterised by progressive replacement of right ventricular myocardium with fatty and fibrous tissue. It is particularly prevalent in young and female patients.

Resting ECG findings in ARVD include T wave inversion in leads V1–V3 with epsilon waves or localised prolongation of the QRS complex (> 0.11 secs or three small squares)

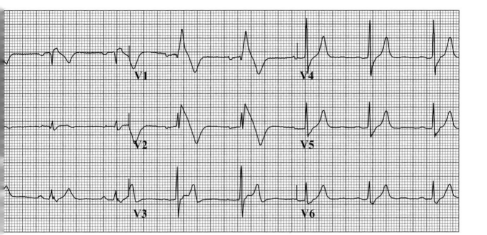

in the right precordial leads. Ambulatory monitoring may reveal frequent ventricular ectopics (greater than 1000 in a 24-hour period) and sustained and non-sustained runs of ventricular tachycardia with a left bundle branch block pattern morphology.

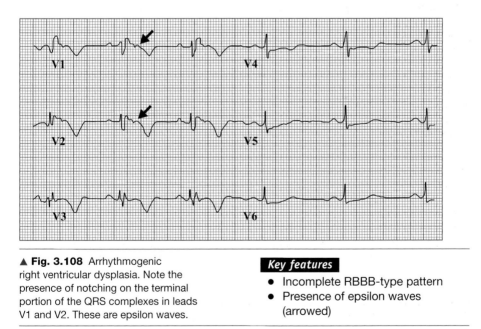

▲ **Fig. 3.108** Arrhythmogenic right ventricular dysplasia. Note the presence of notching on the terminal portion of the QRS complexes in leads V1 and V2. These are epsilon waves.

Key features

- Incomplete RBBB-type pattern
- Presence of epsilon waves (arrowed)

Other causes
Other causes of sudden cardiac death are hypertrophic and dilated cardiomyopathy and idiopathic ventricular fibrillation, a disorder of unknown cause.

TRIFASCICULAR BLOCK

Present when bifascicular block is associated with first degree heart block. A typical ECG would demonstrate right bundle branch block with left or right axis deviation and first degree heart block.

See also:
Bifascicular block
Left anterior hemiblock
Left posterior hemiblock.

WOLF–PARKINSON–WHITE SYNDROME (WPW)

Wolf–Parkinson–White syndrome, named after the three physicians who established it as a clinical entity in 1930, is a congenital cardiac anomaly resulting from incomplete separation of the atria and ventricles during foetal development. Described as the bundle of Kent, the accessory pathway in WPW provides an additional route of conduction between the atria and ventricles.

During sinus rhythm an impulse will be conducted to the ventricles via both the AV node and the accessory pathway. Because conduction through the normal AV node is slower than in the accessory pathway initial ventricular activation is rapid, leading to ventricular pre-excitation, hence the PR interval is short. However, because the accessory pathway is not connected to the specialised conduction system the passage through the initial portion of the ventricular myocardium is slow. This gives rise to the delta wave on the ECG. During sinus rhythm ventricular conduction is a fusion between

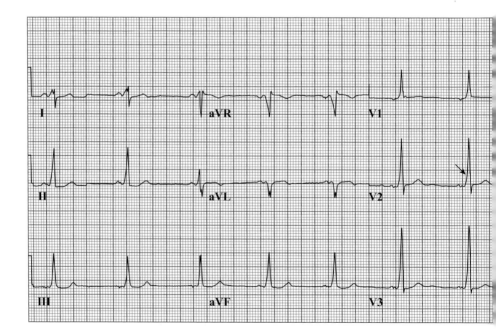

the delta wave and a normally conducted impulse. The presence and direction of the delta wave is influenced by the location of the accessory pathway. It is at this point that WPW falls into two so-called "types": type A and type B.

In WPW type A the delta wave is anteriorly-directed, anatomically-speaking. This typically gives rise to the ECG pattern shown below.

In type A WPW a premature activation occurs in the left ventricle. Superficially type A WPW can mimic right bundle branch block, right ventricular hypertrophy and posterior MI.

In type B WPW the delta wave is directed posteriorly and is less readily distinguished.

Type B WPW may superficially resemble left bundle branch block or an old anteroseptal MI. Premature activation in type B WPW occurs in the right ventricle.

This is the classic characterisation of WPW as it appears on the ECG and in almost all standard texts. However, a word of caution is needed. In practice the PR interval may be longer than 0.12 seconds and the QRS duration nearer to 0.10 seconds. The key, then, is in recognising the presence of a delta wave. Furthermore, classification into these two types is rather an oversimplification – many cases of WPW do not fall into either type A or B. For instance an inferiorly-directed delta wave results in Q or QS waves in leads II, III and aVF and closely resembles an old inferior MI.

However, don't worry too much; it is not the location of the delta wave but rather the potential for re-entry tachycardias via the pathway which is more important and it is the frequent occurrence of supraventricular tachyarrhythmias which is the most significant clinical aspect of WPW syndrome.

The AV re-entry mechanism in WPW is described as being either orthodromic or antidromic. In orthodromic propagation an ectopic atrial impulse is conducted in the normal

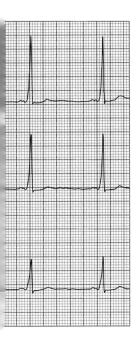

◀ **Fig. 3.109** Wolf–Parkinson–White syndrome type A.

Key features

- Dominant R wave in lead V1
- Short PR interval and delta wave (arrowed)

151

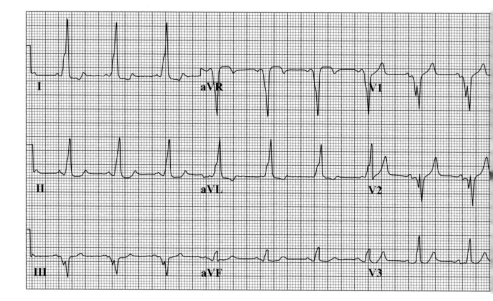

way through the AV node to the ventricles but then in a retrograde fashion from the ventricles to the atria via the accessory pathway. This sets up a self-perpetuating circuit and results in a narrow complex tachycardia with a rate in the region of 140–250 bpm. The P waves during this form of tachycardia are inscribed after the QRS complex and are inverted.

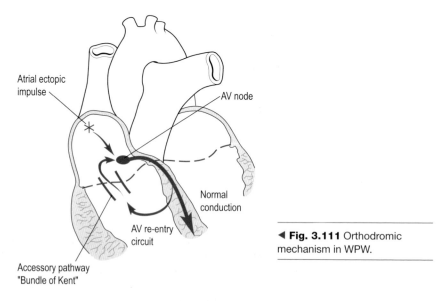

◀ **Fig. 3.111** Orthodromic mechanism in WPW.

Antidromic conduction allows anterograde (or forward) conduction via the accessory pathway from the atria to the ventricles and then retrogradely from the ventricles to the atria via the AV node. Because depolarisation is partially propagated via the ventricular myocardium the resulting QRS appears broad.

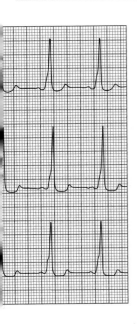

◀ **Fig. 3.110** Wolf–Parkinson–White syndrome type B.

Key features

- Negative QRS complexes and delta waves in leads V1 and V2
- Short PR interval

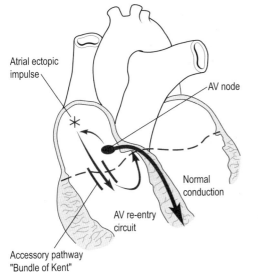

◀ **Fig. 3.112** Antidromic mechanism in WPW.

Atrial flutter and fibrillation in WPW

The incidence of atrial flutter and fibrillation associated with WPW syndrome is as low as 20–25% but can be potentially fatal. In the structurally normal heart the ventricles are protected from excessively high rates by the AV node (remember that atrial flutter and fibrillation can cause atrial contractions in excess of 300 bpm). In patients with an accessory pathway, however, conduction between atria and ventricles can occur in a ratio of 1:1. QRS conduction during these arrhythmias is always broad and bizarre, partly due to the anomalous AV connection and also because these impulses are often aberrantly conducted. Such excessively high ventricular rates can lead to heart failure, ventricular fibrillation and sudden death.

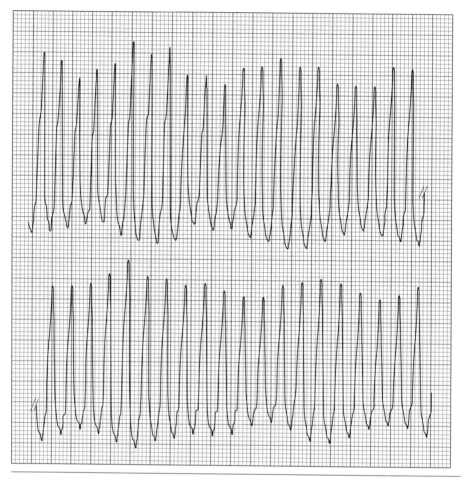

▲ **Fig. 3.113** Atrial fibrillation with WPW. This ECG was recorded from a 23-year-old man who was brought to casualty complaining of palpitations, chest pain and vomiting. On the cardiac monitor, his heart rate was approaching 300 bpm, and BP was 80/50. The patient was sedated urgently, and DC cardioversion was successfully performed.

Key features

- Broad and extremely rapid ventricular activation
- Broad complex QRS

Caution should again be implemented in the treatment of arrhythmias in WPW because agents such as digoxin and verapamil may be dangerous in this situation as they block the AV node and encourage propagation via the accessory pathway. In patients presenting with rapid AF in WPW prompt DC cardioversion must be considered. Drugs that slow anomalous conduction via the accessory pathway are procainamide, amiodarone and quinidine. In patients with re-entry tachycardias in WPW and narrow QRS complexes, adenosine or DC cardioversion is recommended acutely and thereafter treatment for preventing tachycardias include beta blockers, type IA and type III drugs and radio-frequency catheter ablation of the accessory pathway.

INDEX